W0091498

CBS Confident Pharmacy Series

Biochemistry and Clinical Pathology

Third Edition

for First Year Diploma in Pharmacy

(0808) Strictly Based on Syllabus as per ER1991

V.N. Raje M Pharm

Principal
Gourishankar Education Society's
GES College of Pharmacy (D Pharm)
Limb, Satara, Maharashtra

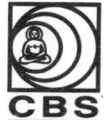

CBS

CBS Publishers & Distributors Pvt Ltd

New Delhi • Bengaluru • Chennai • Kochi • Kolkata • Lucknow • Mumbai
Hyderabad • Jharkhand • Nagpur • Patna • Pune • Uttarakhand

Disclaimer

Science and technology are constantly changing fields. New research and experience broaden the scope of information and knowledge. The author has tried his best in giving information available to him while preparing the material for this book. Although, all efforts have been made to ensure optimum accuracy of the material, yet it is quite possible some errors might have been left uncorrected. The publisher, the printer and the author will not be held responsible for any inadvertent errors or inaccuracies.

Biochemistry and Clinical Pathology

Third Edition

ISBN: 978-93-86478-53-5 ·

Copyright © Author and Publisher

Third Edition: 2018

   Reprint: 2018, 2019, 2020, 2021 2022,

First Edition: 2010

Second Edition: 2015

   Reprint: 2016

All rights reserved. No part of this book may be reproduced or transmitted in any form or by any means, electronic or mechanical, including photocopying, recording, or any information storage and retrieval system without permission, in writing, from the author and the publisher.

Published by Satish Kumar Jain and produced by Varun Jain for

CBS Publishers & Distributors Pvt Ltd

4819/XI Prahlad Street, 24 Ansari Road, Daryaganj, New Delhi 110 002, India.
Ph: 011-23289259, 23266861, 23266867   Website: www.cbspd.com
Fax: 011-23243014   e-mail: delhi@cbspd.com; cbspubs@airteimail.in.
Corporate Office: 204 FIE, Industrial Area, Patparganj, Delhi 110 092

Ph: 011-4934 4934   Fax: 011-4934 4935   e-mail: publishing@cbspd.com;
publicity@cbspd.com

Branches

- **Bengaluru:** Seema House 2975, 17th Cross, K.R. Road, Banasankari 2nd Stage, Bengaluru 560 070, Karnataka
  Ph: +91-80-26771678/79   Fax: +91-80-26771680   e-mail: bangalore@cbspd.com
- **Chennai:** 7, Subbaraya Street, Shenoy Nagar, Chennai 600 030, Tamil Nadu
  Ph: +91-44-26680620, 26681266 Fax: +91-44-42032115   e-mail: chennai@cbspd.com
- **Kochi:** 42/1325, 1326, Power House Road, Opp KSEB, Power House, Ernakulum Kochi 682 018, Kerala, India
  Ph: +91-484-4059061-65,67   Fax: +91-484-4059065   e-mail: kochi@cbspd.com
- **Kolkata:** 147, Hind Ceramics Compound, 1st Floor, Nilgunj Road, Belghoria, Kolkata-700056, West Bengal, India
  Ph: +91-9096713055/7798394118, 9836841399   e-mail: kolkata@cbspd.com
- **Lucknow:** Basement, Khushnuma Complex, 7 Meerabai Marg (Behind Jawahar Bhawan), Lucknow-226001, UP
  Ph: +0522-4000032   e-mail: tiwari.lucknow@cbspd.com
- **Mumbai:** PWD Shed, Gala no 25/26, Ramchandra Bhatt Marg, Next to JJ Hospital Gate no. 2, Opp. Union Bank of India, Noorbaug, Mumbai-400009, Maharashtra, India
  Ph: 022-66661880/89   e-mail: mumbai@cbspd.com

Representatives

- Hyderabad   0-9885175004
- Patna   0-9334159340
- Jharkhand   0-9811541605
- Pune   0-9623451994
- Nagpur   0-9421945513
- Uttarakhand 0-9716462459

Printed at: Mudrak, Noida, UP

CBS Confident Pharmacy Series

Biochemistry and Clinical Pathology

Third Edition

for First Year Diploma in Pharmacy

(0808) Strictly Based on Syllabus as per ER1991

Question–Answer Type Notes and Board Question Papers (1996 to 2017)

Salient Features

- ❏ Total Confidence and 100 percent Success in Every Examination.
- ❏ Repeatedly Asked Board Questions Indicated in Brackets.
- ❏ Chapterwise Collection of Very Important Questions.
- ❏ Written in Very Simple and Lucid Language.
- ❏ Board Question Papers 2015–2017 given at the End of Text.

CBS Titles by the same Author in

CBS Confident Pharmacy Series

First Year D Pharm

1. Pharmaceutics I, 3/e
2. Pharmaceutical Chemistry I, 3/e
3. Pharmacognosy, 3/e
4. Biochemistry and Clinical Pathology, 3/e
5. Human Anatomy and Physiology, 3/e
6. Health Education and Community Pharmacy, 3/e

Second Year D Pharm

1. Pharmaceutics II, 3/e
2. Pharmaceutical Chemistry II, 3/e
3. Pharmacology and Toxicology, 3/e
4. Pharmaceutical Jurisprudence, 3/e
5. Drug Store and Business Management, 3/e
6. Hospital and Clinical Pharmacy, 3/e

to
my beloved family

Preface to the Third Edition

The third edition of the now popular and successful book includes Board Question Papers 1996 to 2017. The book has been written to meet the requirements of students of Diploma in Pharmacy (D Pharm) in accordance with the new revised syllabus ER1991 prescribed by Pharmacy Council of India.

This book is small and humble effort has been put in for compiling necessary information on the subject. An attempt has been made to demystify and simplify the basic concepts for the students of pharmacy and to enable them get an evergreen success in MSBTE examinations.

The salient features of the present book are:

• Lucid and easy language,
• To the point answers,
• Remembering facts in the simplest way, and
• Infusing confidence in the reader to appear in the Board Examinations.

Hence the series is named

CBS Confident Pharmacy Series

I am confident that this book will be useful to both the students and the teachers of Diploma in Pharmacy as well as the candidates desiring to succeed in competitive examinations for better job opportunities in pharmacy profession such as hospital pharmacists in PHCs, civil hospitals, etc.

Raje Vijay N

Acknowledgements

I express my heartfelt thanks to Prof Madan Jagtap, Chairman, Gourishankar Education Society, Satara Maharashtra, for consistent encouragement and inspiration for writing this book.

I wish to acknowledge the prompt and efficient help given by Prof Milind Jagtap, Mr Jaywant Salunkhe, Mr Appa Rajage, Mr Nitin Mudalgikar, and Mr Shrirang Katekar of Gourishankar Education Society, Satara.

I am also thankful to Shri Satish Kumar Jain, Chairman and Managing Director, and Shri RN Mandal, General Manager, Pune Branch, CBS Publishers & Distributors Pvt Ltd, for their sustained efforts and keen interest in the publication of this book.

I wish all my beloved students to have a great success in the Board Examinations.

Raje Vijay N

Syllabus

(As per ER 1991)

Biochemistry and Clinical Pathology

1. Introduction to Biochemistry
2. Brief chemistry and role of proteins, polypeptides and amino acids, classification, qualitative tests, biological value, Deficiency disease.
3. Brief chemistry and role of carbohydrates, classification qualitative tests. Diseases related to carbohydrate metabolism
4. Brief chemistry and role of lipids, classification, qualitative tests, Diseases related to lipid metabolism
5. Brief chemistry and role of vitamins and coenzymes
6. Role of minerals and water in life processes
7. Enzymes: Brief concept of enzymic action factors affecting it. Therapeutic and pharmaceutical importance
8. Brief concept of normal and abnormal metabolism of proteins, carbohydrates and lipids.
9. Introduction to pathology of blood and urine
   a. Lymphocytes and platelets, their role in health and diseases.
   b. Erythrocytes—Abnormal cells and their significance
   c. Abnormal constituents of urine and their significance in diseases.

Contents

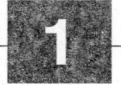

Introduction to Biochemistry

Q 1. Define the terms: (S. 96, 97, 02, 03, 04; W. 01, 05, 08)

a. *Biochemistry*: Biochemistry is the study of chemistry of living organism and deals with structure of tissues, cells, organelles and individual biomolecules.

b. *The cell*: The cell is the basic, living, structural and functional unit of living organism.

c. *Biomolecules*: The living cell is composed of few elements like C, H, O and N that combine to form a great variety of molecules are called as biomolecules, e.g. carbohydrates, proteins, fats, nucleic acids, lipids.

Q 2. Give the aims, objectives, importance of biochemistry. (W. 01)

i. Biochemistry is helpful for detail study of structure and functions of biomolecules like carbohydrates, proteins, lipids, minerals and DNA.

ii. Biochemistry is useful for study of various interactions of different biomolecules.

iii. Biochemistry is useful for study of nature and working of enzymes and study of different types of enzymes.

iv. Study of the energy transformations in living cells, organisms is another objective of study of biochemistry.

v. Heredity and variations, possess rational molecular basis. The study of this molecular basis is one of the main aim of biochemistry.

vi. Study of self-replication and duplication processes which maintains the genetic continuity from cell to cell, is main objective of biochemistry.

vii. Knowledge of biochemistry is used to control diseases, abnormal deficiency and treatment of deficiencies.

viii. Metabolic abnormalities can be studied by the knowledge of biochemistry.

ix. Knowledge of biochemistry is helpful for understanding the dynamic changes of cellular systems and corresponding need of nutrients.

Q 3. Discuss major intracellular organ and their functions. OR Describe various parts of cell, draw and label diagram of cell. (S. 98, 05, 06, 07, 08; W. 03)

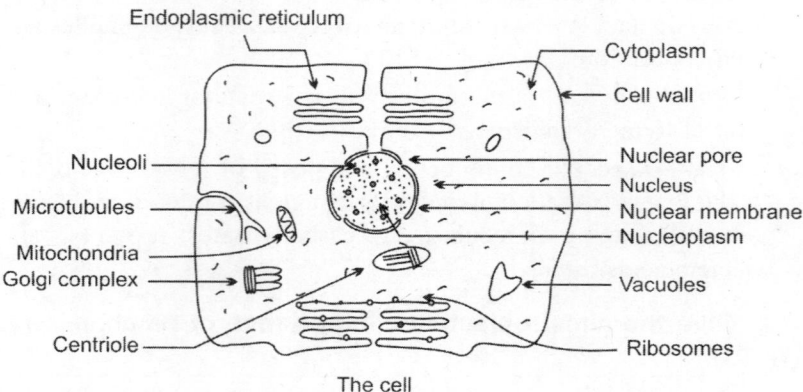

The cell

Parts /Components of Cell/Major Intracellular Organs/Organelles

1. *Nucleus*: It is spherical and largest part of the cell. It contains nuclear membrane, nucleoplasm, nucleoli and genetic material DNA. Nuclear membrane is continuous with endoplasmic reticulum.
   - *Functions*:
     i. It controls all cellular activities.
     ii. It contains DNA, RNA and proteins.
     iii. RNA helps in protein synthesis.
     iv. DNA helps in production of chromosomes.
     v. Marker enzyme is DNA polymerase which is a site of DNA to RNA synthesis.
2. *Endoplasmic reticulum*: It is a network of membrane continuous with nuclear membrane.

- *Functions*:
  - i. It provides surface area for number of chemical reactions.
  - ii. It helps in synthesis of a steroids, protein, etc.
  - iii. It provides a pathway for transporting various chemical substances.
  - iv. It helps to concentrate the products of synthetic activities of cell.

3. *Ribosomes*: These are tiny granules present in cytoplasm as well as on surface of endoplasmic reticulum. It contains special type of RNA called RNA.
   - *Function:* Ribosomes are the main sites for protein synthesis.

4. *Lysosome*: These are membranous vesicles contains powerful digestive enzymes which are capable of breaking down many kinds of molecules.
   - *Functions*:
     - i. It helps for intracellular digestion
     - ii. Autolysis
     - iii. Phagocytosis.

5. *Golgi apparatus*: It consists of 4 to 8 flattened bag like channels stacked upon each other. It is located near the nucleus.
   - *Functions*:
     - i. It helps in intracellular sorting of proteins
     - ii. It helps in packaging of secretory products.

6. *Mitochondria (S. 96, W. 98, 01, 04, 05)*: There are small intracellular organelles and are known as power house of cells. It is bounded by inner folded and other smooth membrane. Inner surface have many cristae and are covered with F_1 particles.
   - *Functions*:
     - i. It is the main site for synthesis and storage of ATP.
     - ii. It is the site of citric acid cycle, β-oxidation, urea cycle, ETS.
     - iii. It contains special DNA and is self-replicative.
     - iv. Mitochondrion performs the main function of conversion and transfer of cellular energy.

7. *Cell membrane/plasma membrane*: It surrounds the cell and separate it from other cells and external environment. It is composed of proteins, phospholipids, carbohydrates, minerals, etc.

- *Functions:*
    i. It involves in transport of molecules in and out of the cells.
    ii. It gives shape to the cell.
    iii. It covers and protects the cell and organelles.
    iv. It helps in intracellular adhesion and communication.
    v. It forms channels of ER.
    vi. It forms boundaries to the cytoplasm.
    vii. It can acts as a physiological sieve.

2

Water and Mineral Metabolism

Q 1. Define and classify minerals with suitable examples. (S. 96, 97, 98, 01, 02, 03, 05, 06; W. 96, 97, 02, 08)

Minerals

Minerals are the elements which are necessary for a variety of physiological functions and number of biochemical processes.

Classification of Minerals

Macrominerals/Macroelements/Principle Elements

The minerals which are required in large quantities for the human body with respect to daily requirement are called as macronutrients, e.g. Ca, P, Na, K, Mg, Fe, Zn, etc.

Microelements/Microminerals/Trace Elements

The minerals which are required in very less quantities (trace quantities) for the human body with respect to daily requirements are called as micronutrients/trace elements, e.g. Co, Cu, I, Se, Mn, etc.

Q 2. Give the functions of minerals in life process. (S. 96, 97, 98, 01, 02, 03, 05, 09; W. 96, 97, 02, 05)

- For maintenance of osmotic pressure of blood (Na^+, K^+, Cl^-)
- For transport of oxygen (Fe)
- For growth and maintenance of tissues and bones (Ca^{++})
- For working of nervous system (Ca^{++})
- For muscle contraction (Ca^{++})
- For maintenance of electrolyte balance (Na^+ K^+)
- For acid–base balance (Na^+)
- For blood coagulation (Ca^{++})
- For cardiac activity (Ca^{++})

- For maturation of sperms (Zn)
- For thyroid hormone synthesis (iodine).

Q 3. Name the conditions after increase and decreased level of following.

Minerals/Sub.	Increased blood level	Decreased blood level
Sodium	Hypernatremia	Hyponatremia
Potassium	Hyperkalemia	Hypokalemia
Chlorine	Hyperchloremia	Hypochloremia
Calcium	Hypercalcemia	Hypocalcemia
Sugar	Hyperglycemia	Hypoglycemia

Q 4. Give the biochemical role (functions) and deficiency disorders of following minerals.

Minerals	Functions/biochemical roles	Deficiency disorders
Calcium (S. 96, 02, 03; W. 97, 98, 00, 02)	i. For formation, maintenance and growth of bones ii. For formation of tooth iii. For blood clotting iv. For absorption of vitamin B_{12} v. For contraction of muscle vi. For activation of enzymes vii. For excitability of nerve fibres	• Rickets • Osteoporosis • Hypocalcemia • Osteomalacia • Tetany
Iron (S. 97, 00, 01; W. 97, 01, 02)	i. For formation of Hb/RBCs ii. For DNA synthesis iii. For formation of myoglobin iv. As an electron carrier v. For transport of gases (O_2 and CO_2)	• Iron deficiency anemia • Hemochromatosis
Iodine	i. For biosynthesis of thyroid hormones ii. For growth and development of body	• Goitre/Goiter • Hypothyroidism • Cretinism
Copper (S. 98)	i. In haemoglobin synthesis ii. For melanin formation	• Homeostasis • Hypochromic

Contd.

Minerals	Functions/biochemical roles	Deficiency disorders
	iii. In bone formation iv. In several enzymes systems v. In maintenance of integrity of myelin sheath	• Microcytic anemia
Phosphorus (S. 98; W. 02)	i. For formation and development of bones and teeth ii. For formation of phospholipids, nucleic acids iii. It forms co-enzymes like NADP, ADP, AMP, ATP iv. It is required in the absorption of glucose by phosphorylation	• Hypophosphatemia • Rickets • Osteomalacia
Sodium	i. For maintenance of osmotic pressure ii. For retaining water in the body iii. For neuromuscular junction activity iv. For excitability of nerves v. For acid–base balance vi. For maintenance of viscosity of blood vii. To maintain electrolyte balance	• Hyponatremia
Potassium (S. 99, 01)	i. For acid–base balance ii. For cardiac function iii. As a co-factor iv. For neuromuscular junction activity v. To neutralize effect of Ca^{++} vi. To maintain osmotic pressure	• Hypokalemia
Chlorine	i. For acid–base balance ii. For secretion of HCl in stomach iii. For maintenance of osmotic pressure iv. For synthesis of CSF	• Hypochloremia

Q 5. What do you mean by 'hypothyroidism' and 'hyperthyroidism'? OR Give the effect of 'hypothyroidism' and 'hyperthyroidism'. (S. 01)

1. *Hypothyroidism*: The decreased secretion of thyroid hormones results into condition called as hypothyroidism.
   - *Effects/symptoms/characteristics of hypothyroidism*:
     i. Slow metabolic processes
     ii. Stunted growth
     iii. Mental retardation
     iv. Low body temperature
     v. Swelling of muscles of face
     vi. Enlargement of thyroid gland
     vii. Swelling of neck.

2. *Hyperthyroidism*: Excessive secretion of thyroid hormones result into hyperthyroidism.
   - *Effects/symptoms*:
     i. Increased BMR
     ii. Increased heart rate
     iii. Anxiety
     iv. Restlessness
     v. Increased blood iodine level
     vi. Increased blood pressure.

Q 6. Explain the terms:

1. *Rickets (S. 98, 05; W. 04)*: It is the disorder common in children. It is caused due to initial deficiency of vitamin D_3 followed by calcium deficiency.
   - *Symptoms/characteristics/effects*:
     i. Demineralization of bones
     ii. Diffused bone pains
     iii. Weak arms and legs
     iv. Skeletal deformity
     v. Muscular weakness
     vi. Bending of bones of arms and legs.

2. *Osteoporosis (S. 03; W. 04)*: It is a disorder common in elder persons. The main cause is reduction in total bone calcium and bones become more fragile.

- *Symptoms*:
    - i. Demineralization of bones
    - ii. Porosity developed in bones
    - iii. Diffused bone pains
    - iv. Pains in the spine
    - v. Bending of thoracic vertebrae
    - vi. Vertebral compression.

3. *Osteomalacia*: It is a calcium deficiency disorder found in adult. It may be due to less intake of calcium or calcium loss in renal failure.

    - *Symptoms*:
        - i. Softening of bones
        - ii. Abnormal development of bones
        - iii. Diffused bone pains
        - iv. Inability of a person to perform sustained work.

4. *Tetany*: Tetany is a disease that occurs due to decreased ionized fraction of serum calcium.

    - *Causes*:
        - i. An increase in pH of blood
        - ii. Poor absorption of calcium from the intestine
        - iii. Decreased dietary intake of calcium
        - iv. Increased renal excretion of calcium
        - v. Increased retention of phosphorus.

    - *Symptoms*:
        - i. Muscles loose tonicity
        - ii. Affects face, hands and feet.

5. *Anemia*: It means an abnormal decrease in haemoglobin or RBCs.

    - *Causes*:
        - i. Excessive blood loss
        - ii. Abnormal menstruation
        - iii. Internal ulcer and bleeding
        - iv. Bleeding from piles
        - v. Intestinal damage
        - vi. Failure of function of bone marrow.

    - *Symptoms*:
        - i. Decreased Hb content

    ii. Low RBC count

    iii. Abnormal structure of RBCs (microcytic)

    iv. Loss of appetite

    v. Breathlessness and restlessness

    vi. Pale skin.

6. *Goitre/goiter* (*S. 08*): It is caused by deficiency of iodine in the blood. Iodine is required for the formation of thyroxine and triiodothyronine.

    • *Symptoms*:

      i. Enlargement of thyroid gland

      ii. Low BMR

      iii. Low pulse rate and heart rate

      iv. Hypotension (low BP)

      v. Metabolic disturbances

      vi. Low body temperature.

    • *Treatment*:

      i. Regular use of iodised salt

      ii. Iodine is added to drinking water.

7. *Hypokalaemia* (*S. 05*): It is an abnormal condition indicating decreased level of potassium in the blood plasma.

    • *Causes*:

      i. Prolonged diarrhoea and vomiting

      ii. Overactivity of adrenal cortex

      iii. Prolonged use of diuretics

      iv. Heart failure treatment with digitalis

      v. Diabetic coma treatment with insulin.

    • *Symptoms*:

      i. Muscular weakness

      ii. Irritability

      iii. Paralysis

      iv. Tachycardia (increased in heart rate)

      v. Dilation of heart

      vi. Changes in ECG.

8. *Hyperkalaemia*: It is an abnormal condition indicating increased level of potassium in blood plasma.

    • *Causes*:

      i. Renal failure

      ii. Severe dehydration

    iii. Excess use of potassium salts by IV

    iv. Shock.

- *Symptoms*:

    i. Cardiac and CNS depression

    ii. Bradycardia

    iii. Peripheral vascular collapse

    iv. Mental confusion

    v. Weakness of respiratory muscles.

9. *Hyponatraemia*: It is an abnormal condition indicating decreased level of Na^+ in blood plasma.

- *Causes*:

    i. Fluid loss from the body

    ii. Kidney failure

    iii. Renal diseases

    iv. Severe burns

    v. Excessive vomiting and diarrhoea

    vi. Prolonged diabetes with polyuria

    vii. Addisions disease.

Q 7. Write a note on "dehydration" (abnormal metabolism of water).

Dehydration

Dehydration is defined as more loss of water from the human body, than the normal output with respect to the input of water.

- *Causes/reasons of dehydration*:

    i. Severe diarrhoea and vomiting due to viral or bacterial infections produce increased water loss causing dehydration.

    ii. De to severe diarrhoea.

    iii. Excess loss of water through expired air may results in certain loss of water causing dehydration.

    iv. The person following desert travel suffer from dehydration.

    v. Mental patients refusing to drink water can cause dehydration.

    vi. The disturbance in exchange of electrolytes during elimination may leads to dehydration.

    vii. In diabetic patients because of body physiology there is an excess of urination, may leads to dehydration.

    viii. Unconscious condition or difficulty in swallowing condition there is a decreased intake of water causing dehydration.

    ix. Unavailability of water for shipwrecked persons cause dehydration.

    x. Loss of water from serious burned cases causes dehydration.

- *Symptoms/characteristics/effects of dehydration*:
  i. Dry and hot skin and dry tongue.
  ii. Very little secretion of tears and saliva.
  iii. Loss of weight due to reduction in tissue water.
  iv. Disturbances in acid–base balance.
  v. Rise in body temperature during reduction in circulating fluid.
  vi. Dryness, wrinkling and loosening of skin.
  vii. Rise in the nonprotein content of plasma.
  viii. Decrease in urine output comparatively.
  ix. Incresed pulse rate and reduced cardiac output.
  x. Much increase in packed cell volume.

- *Treatments of dehydration*:
  i. By giving plenty of water as oral drinks.
  ii. IV administration of fluids.
  iii. Dextrose saline as energy.
  iv. Keep the victim in a cool environment.

Q 8. State the 'properties of water'. What is the biological role of water? (S. 98, 01, 03; W. 96, 97, 03)

Properties of Water

    i. Water can dissociate in the hydronium and hydroxy ion.

$$H_2O \longrightarrow H^+ + OH^-$$

    ii. Water is capable of interacting with many inorganic or organic molecules such as proteins, sugar, etc.

    iii. Water helps to maintain characteristic structure and specific biological properties of proteins, nucleic acids and ATP.

    iv. Specific heat of water is much high hence it can work as a best medium for absorption of heat.

    v. Water has very high dielectric constant.

    vi. Water is a polar molecule, due to which water is very good solvent.

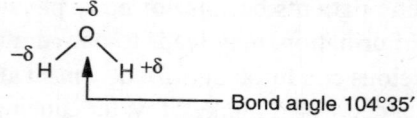

Bond angle 104°35′

Biological Role of Water

i. Water can acts as best transportation medium in the body.

ii. Water act as a best solvent for different organic and inorganic substances.

iii. Water dissociates into H^+ and OH^- and act as a hydrogen donor for various metabolic reactions.

iv. Water is highly inert and simplest in chemical nature. Hence, it can participate in variety of biochemical reactions.

v. Water helps to maintain constant body temperature.

vi. Water is a polar molecule, it can take part in different biochemical reactions.

vii. Water dissociate into hydrogen ion (H^+), which maintains the pH of the body, and is essential for activity of enzymes in biological system.

viii. Water interact with various substances and provides specific properties to the cell.

ix. Dehydration of rehydration are specific reactions related with water as a part of many metabolic pathways.

x. Water can interact with many substances like proteins, fats, carbohydrates and keep them in biological functional form.

Q 9. Explain water balance in our body. Give the mechanism of balancing body water content. Describe regulation of water content in human body. (S. 96, 02, 03, 04, 07, 08; W. 02, 03, 04)

Water is most common and abundant compound of all living system. An equilibrium is maintained between intake and loss of water from the body. The regulation of water balance is influenced by certain hormones such as ADH, aldosterone, etc.

The specific ways of intake and output of water with corresponding are showing below figures (in normal healthy adult).

Water input		Water output	
1. Oral drinks	1200 ml	1. Urination	1400 ml
2. Solid food	1000 ml	2. Sweating	600 ml
3. Oxidation of food stuff	300 ml	3. Expiration	300 ml
Total input	2500 ml	4. Defecation	200 ml
		Total output	2500 ml

Mechanism of Balancing Body Water Content

Thirst Mechanism

The decreased in water content of the body leads to dehydration. This stimulates the sensory nerves in mouth and tongue and shows sensation of feeling of thirst. Thus individual drinks water. Thus, water content of the body is balanced with respect to input and outputs.

Urine Output Mechanism/ADH Mechanism

This is the another mechanism to balance body water content. When water content in the body is less, then blood get concentrated. This decreases osmotic pressure of blood. So osmoreceptor of kidneys are stimulated and this information is given to the brain (hypothalamus) by sensory nerves. The posterior lobe of pituitary gland stimulates and release ADH (anti-diuretic hormone). This hormone increases reabsorption of water from urinary filtrate and water content in body is balanced.

Water content less

↓

Osmotic pressure of blood decreases

↓

Stimulates osmoreceptor of kidney

↓

Information given to hypothalamus

↓

Stimulates posterior pituitary gland

↓

ADH secretion

↓

Increased reabsorption of water from filtrate

↓

Water level increases

↓

Effect of ADH inhibited

3

Proteins

Q 1. What are proteins? Classify proteins with suitable examples. (S.96, 06, 09; W. 98, 01, 03)

Proteins

Proteins are naturally occurring polymers made up of amino acids linked together by peptide bonds (–CONH–) having high molecular weight found in all living cells.

Classification of Proteins

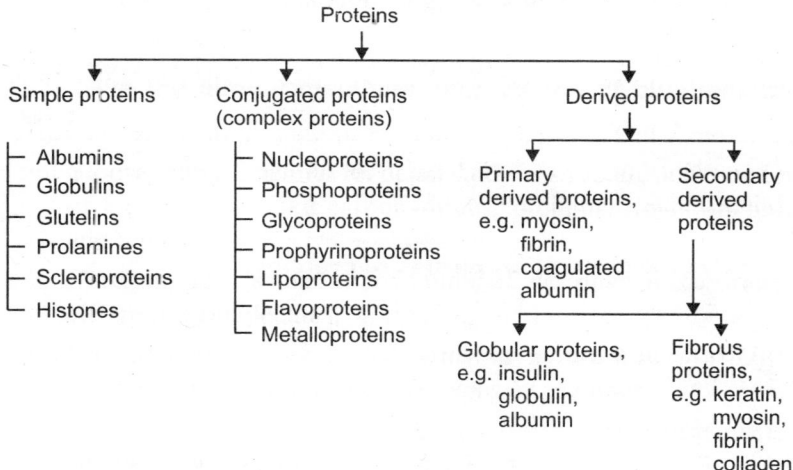

Q 2. What do you mean by "complete proteins" and "incomplete proteins"? Give example. (S. 00)

Complete Proteins

"The proteins which contains all essential amino acids in required quantities are called as complete protein," e.g. milk proteins, egg proteins.

Incomplete Proteins

"The proteins not containing all essential amino acids are called as incomplete proteins," e.g. gelatin, zein of maize.

Q 3. Give biological importance/functions of proteins. (S. 97, 00, 01, 08; W. 96, 97, 99, 03, 07, 08)

- Proteins are the essence of life process.
- Proteins are important for the structures of membrane muscular tissue or connective tissues.
- Nucleoproteins have a great significance in genetics.
- Number of enzymes are proteins which catalyze number of biochemical reactions.
- Proteins are important for transport of oxygen throughout the body, e.g. haemoglobin.
- Proteins maintains the fluid balance.
- Proteins are important in regulation of metabolism by hormones such as insulin and glucagon.
- Proteins are responsible for protection against infection and other toxic substances.
- Proteins which are required to carry-out mechanical work are called as muscle protein, e.g. myosin.
- Proteins which are required to give strength to the cells or tissues of the body called as structural proteins, e.g. lipoproteins, phosphoproteins, collagen.

Q 4. State the general properties of proteins.

1. *Solubility*: Some proteins are soluble in water and some are soluble in weak salt solution, acid and alkalies. Some proteins are soluble in organic solvents like acetone chloroform. Proteins generally forms colloidal solution.
2. *Precipitation*: Proteins are precipitated by salt of heavy metals, like mercury, tungsten, silver, etc.
3. *Amphoteric nature*: Proteins are made up of amino acids which are amphoteric, i.e. posses equal negative and positive charges.
4. *Coagulation*: Protein are heat sensitive, so they can be coagulated by applying heat, where peptide bonds are broken and coagulates proteins.

5. *Colour reactions*: Almost all proteins give certain coloured reaction positive when treated with specific reagents. Hence, helpful in laboratory diagnosis.

6. *Molecular weight*: Proteins have very high molecular weight ranges between few thousands to one millions or more.

7. *Protein hydrolysis*: Proteins can be hydrolysed to obtain respective constituent as amino acids and nonprotein compound.

Q 5. Give the coloured reactions/qualitative test for proteins and amino acids.

1. *Xanthoproteic test* (*S. 01; W. 00*): Proteins when treated with concentration HNO_3 produce deep yellow or orange colour, upon addition of alkali.

   - *Principle*: Aromatic amino acids like phenyl alanine, tyrosine gives this coloured reaction positive. In actual reaction particular amino acid reacts with HNO_3 to form metaproteins. Nitrocompounds actually develop deep yellow orange colour. Such colour is produced in alkaline medium because nitrocompounds undergo ionisation in alkaline medium only.

2. *Sakaguchi test* (*test for arginine*) (*W. 00*): Proteins containing amino acid arginine, when boiled with Sakaguchi reagent (reagent containing sodium hypochlorite in α-naphthol) produce red or deep red colour.

   - *Principle*: Arginine in presence of alcoholic α-naphthol forms complex with sodium hypochlorite to produce particular red or deep red coloured conjugate.

3. *Millions reagent test* (*test for tyrosine*) (*S. 97; W. 00*): Proteins containing amino acid tyrosine when treated with millions reagent (mercuric sulphate in acidic medium with sodium nitrite) produce red colour or red coloured precipitate.

   - *Principle*: Amino acid tyrosine with acidified mercury sulphate forms red phenolic complex of the mercury to produce specific red colour or red coloured pecipitate. For protein gelatin this test is positive because of absence of tyrosine in gelatin.

4. *Ninhydrin reaction/test* (*S. 96, 99, 02, 03; W. 96, 98*): Proteins containing ninhydrin compound give this reaction positive producing blue colour upon heating.

- *Principle*: Free amino group of protein or polypeptide or amino acid reacts with ninhydrin reagent to produce specific blue colour, where heating is required.
- *Significance*:
  - i. This test is used to indicate the presence of proteins, polypeptides, peptides and amino acids.
  - ii. Derived proteins like proteases and peptones are also detected.
  - iii. This test is of preliminary importance in laboratory detection of proteins.

5. *Nitroprusside test (test of cystine)*: Cystine or protein containing cystine produce red colour when treated with sodium nitroprusside in dilute NaOH solution.

   In alkaline condition cystine (sulphur containing amino acid) interact with sodium nitroprusside to produce red colour.

6. *Biuret test (S. 98, 01; W. 01)*: It is the test given positive by all compounds containing more than one peptide linkage, i.e. given positive by proteins, proteoses, peptones and polypeptides till tripeptide.

   This test is also positive for substances which contain (–CO–NH$_2$) group.

   - *Principle*: In actual test dilute CuSO$_4$ solution (1%) reacts with protein in alkaline medium, to produce violet or deep violet colour. Medium in test tube is made alkaline by 40% NaOH solution. The specific colour is produced due to formation of copper complexes which indicates actually the presence of peptide linkages.
   - *Significance*: This test possess significance in laboratory detection of proteins and differentiating them from any other organic compound which does not posses peptide linkage.

7. *Hoffkins cole reaction/test*: Protein containing amino acid tryptophan give this test positive producing violet or purple coloured ring at junction of two liquids.

   - *Principle*: Solution containing protein upon reaction with Hoffkins cole reagent (glyoxillic aid) upon addition of concentration H$_2$SO$_4$ very slowly from the sides of test tube from two separate layers producing violet or purple colour at the junction of two liquids.

8. *Heat coagulation test*: Take the test solution of protein up to 2/3rd of the test tube and heat the upper portion of the solution holding the lower part of the test tube.

An opalescence appear which becomes deep upon addition of few drops of 2% acetic acid.

This indicate the presence of proteins (albumin).

Q 6. What are amino acids? Classify with examples. Given biological importance of amino acids. (S. 98, 01, 07; W. 96, 97, 98, 02, 03, 05)

Amino Acid

Amino acid are the monomers of proteins having an amino and carboxyl group attached to the same carbon atom.

General Structure

$$R-\overset{\overset{\displaystyle H}{|}}{\underset{\underset{\displaystyle NH_2}{|}}{C}}-COOH \quad\text{——————— (Acid)}$$
$$\alpha \quad\quad\quad\quad\quad\text{——————— (Amino)}$$

Classification of Amino Acids

i. Amino acid are classified into three groups:
   - *Neutral amino acids*: Glycine, alanine, valine, leucine, serine.
   - *Basic amino acids*: Lysine, arginine, histidine.
   - *Acidic amino acids*: Aspartic acid, glutamic acid, glycine, alanine, valine, leucine, serine.

ii. Amino acid can be classified in another fashion:
   - *Aliphatic amino acids*: Glycine, alanine.
   - *Aromatic amino acids*: Phenyl alanine, tyrosine, tryptophan.
   - *Sulphur amino acids*: Cysteine, methionine.

iii. According to dietary value:
   - *Essential amino acids*: Leucine, isoleucine, arginine.
   - *Nonessential amino acids*: Alanine, glycine, tyrosine.

Biological Role/Functions/Importance/Significance of Amino Acids

i. Amino acids are required for synthesis of various enzymes, hormones, plasma proteins and immunoglobulins.

ii. For growth and repair of body tissues.

iii. As a source of energy when body is having in adequate supply of carbohydrate or fat.

iv. Metabolic products of certain amino acids provides source for energy.

v. Glycine and glutamic acid are involved in the transmission of impulses in the nervous system.

Q 7. Define 'essential and nonessential amino acids' with examples: (S. 96, 97, 98, 01, 02, 03, 07, 09; W. 99, 01, 05, 07, 08)

- *Essential amino acid*: The amino acids which cannot be synthesized in the body, but are badly required for normal functioning are called essential amino acids. For example, leucine, isoleucine, arginine, histidine, valine, phenylalanine.

- *Nonessential amino acid*: The amino acids which can be synthesized in the body but are not very essential for normal functioning of the body are called nonessential amino acids. For example, alanine, glycine, tyrosine, cystine, proline, glutamic acid.

Q 8. Explain physical properties of amino acids. (W. 99, 00, 02)

Properties of Amino Acids

1. *Solubility*:
   - All amino acids are soluble in water but their solubility varies to great extent.
   - Polar amino acids are highly soluble in water.
   - Nonpolar amino acids are highly soluble in organic solvents like alcohol, chloroform, ether, etc.

2. *Optical activity*: Except glycine all amino acids are optically active due to presence of asymmetric carbon atom.

3. *Acid-base behaviour of amino acids (S. 96, 04, 05, 06; W. 98, 01, 02, 07)*: Amino acids contain the acidic group carboxyl (–COOH) and the basic group amino (–NH$_2$). Hence amino acids are amphoteric in nature. Ionisation of there groups depend upon pH of the system and nature of R-group of amino acids.

   - *Isoelectric pH*: The pH at which amino acid carries zero net charge is called as isoelectric pH.

     At an isoelectric pH pure amino acid exist as dipolar ion, i.e. zwitterion. Amino acid zwitterion form possess equal positive and negative electric charge, i.e. net charge zero. The ionisation behaviour of amino acids can be shown as follows:

COOH		$COO^{\ominus}$		$COO^{\ominus}$
$+H_3N$ —— C —— H	$\xrightarrow{\oplus}$	H_3N —— C —— H	$\longrightarrow$	$+H_2N$ —— C —— H
R	$\oplus H$	R	$H\oplus$	R
(Cationic)		(Zwitterion)		(Anionic)

Thus amino acids are positively charged at extreme acidic pH and negatively charged at extreme alkaline pH. There exists an intermediate pH at which net charge of amino acid is zero. At such isoelectric pH amino acids are quite insoluble in water and so they can be precipitated out. This is called isoelectric precipitation of amino acids.

Isoelectric pH can be calculated by formula,

$$I^{pH} = \frac{p^{K_1} + p^{K_2}}{2}$$

where, I^{pH} = Isoelectric pH

p^{K_1} = Negative log of dissociation constant of carboxylic group.

p^{K_2} = Negative log of dissociation constant of amino group.

Q 9. Write a note on "denaturation of proteins". (S. 03, 04; W. 02, 07)

Denaturation of Proteins

"The breakdown of secondary, tertiary and quaternary structure of native proteins resulting in the alterations of the physical, chemical and biological characteristic of protein by a variety of agents."

Denaturation of proteins can be done by following agents:

i. Physical agents, e.g. heat, surface action, UV light, high pressure.

ii. Chemical agents, e.g. acid, alkalies, heavy metal salt, urea.

iii. Biological agents, e.g. proteolytic enzymes.

Changes Occur During Denaturation of Proteins

i. *Physical change*: Many proteins especially globular type can be crystallized in native state but denatured proteins can not be crystallized.

ii. *Chemical change*: The denatured proteins shows decreased solubility.

iii. *Biological change*: Enzymatic and hormonary activity is usually destroyed by denaturation.

Significance

   i. Precipitation of proteins by denaturation helps in clinical laboratory.
  ii. Blood and serum samples are easily analysed by removing protein fraction.
 iii. To check the loss of enzymatic activity when boiled or acidified.

Q 10. What are peptides and polypeptides? Give its biological importance. (S. 98; W. 97, 99)

Peptide

A peptide consist of two or more amino acids linked by a peptide bond (–CONH–) formed be the carboxyl group of one amino acid and amino group of another amino acid with the removal of one molecule of water.

When two amino acids combine in this way, the resultant product is dipeptide. When three amino acids combine, produce tripeptide, when four amino acids combines produce tetrapeptide and many amino acids forms polypeptides.

Proteins are the polypeptides containing at least 100 or more amino acids but there is no clear dividing line both polypeptide and proteins.

Biological Importance of Peptides and Polypeptides

   i. Insulin is a peptide and plays importance role in glucose metabolism.

α-amino acid   α-amino acid   Peptide bond

  ii. Valinomycin and gramicidine are peptides useful as antibiotics.
 iii. Bleomycin, a peptide used as anticancer agent.
  iv. Bradykinin is a polypeptide used as hypotensive agent.
   v. TRH (thyrotropin releasing hormone) is a peptide.

Q 11. Describe the structure of proteins. (S. 96, 00; W. 97, 99, 01)

The structure of protein can be studied as follows:

1. Primary structure
2. Secondary structure
3. Tertiary structure
4. Quaternary structure

1. Primary Structure of Protein (W. 05)

Primary structure of protein means simply a polypeptide chain. It includes the study of sequence of amino acids in proteins. Peptide bonds are the most common linkages involved in formation of primary structure of protein. All amino acids linked together in primary structure are in one plane. Peptide bond is formed by the amino acid linked by carboxyl group of one amino acid with amino group of another amino acid.

The primary structure ultimately becomes as:

$$\overset{\displaystyle R}{\underset{\displaystyle |}{}} \qquad \overset{\displaystyle R}{\underset{\displaystyle |}{}}$$
$$—COOH—CH—\overset{}{\underset{}{}}CONH\overset{}{\underset{}{}}—CH—$$

Peptide linkage

2. Secondary Structure of Proteins (S. 04, 06, 07; W. 03, 07, 08)

Secondary structure of protein is determined by specific geometric arrangements of polypeptide chain.

There arrangements are due to hydrogen bonding between amino group and carbonyl oxygen of peptide bonds. This is called as the secondary structure of proteins.

Three types of secondary structures are possible:

i.   *α-helix structure*: In this case the polypeptide chain twists into a right hand side so that hydrogen bond is formed between C=O and NH, e.g. hair protein, i.e. keratin is made up of α-helix only.

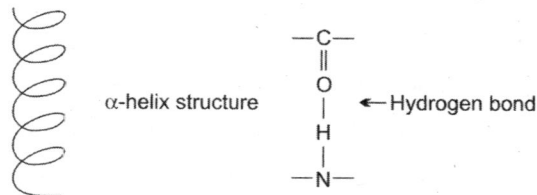

ii. *β-pleated structure of protein*: Here 2 polypeptide chains are present in a structure. There polypeptide chains lying side by side and can form hydrogen bonds between C=O and NH group of neighbouring polypeptide chain. Along with 'H' group of neighbouring polypeptide chain. Alongwith 'H' bonds, disulphide linkages are also formed. Keep two polypeptide chains away at specific distance. Such structure of protein appears like pleated sheet. So it is called β-pleated sheet.

iii. *Reverse turn structure*: The polypeptide chain may be folded back in itself to change or even reverse the direction of chain.

3. Tertiary Structure of Proteins

The peptide chain with coiled secondary structure may get further folded to from 3-D conformation giving rise to tertiary structure. It is stable final structural form, which decides and governs biological and functional properties of that particular protein. Different types of forces/bonds involved in the formation of stable tertiary structure of proteins are as follows:

   i. Vander waals forces
  ii. Electrostatic forces of alteration
 iii. Hydrogen bonds
 iv. Hydrophobic interactions
  v. Disulphide bonds.

4. Quaternary Structure of Proteins

Some proteins contain two or more polypeptides held together by noncovalent interaction. They are called quaternary proteins, e.g. haemoglobin, myoglobin.

It has four subunit. Two alpha and two beta polypeptide chain each has a tertiary structure similar to myoglobin.

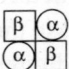

Quarternary structure of proteins

Q 12. Explain any three protein deficiency disorders. (S. 06)

Protein Deficiency Disorders

1. *Kwashiorkor disease (S. 00, 01, 04, 05; W. 04)*

It is a protein deficiency disease occurring commonly in the children. It is characterized by qualitative and quantitative deficiency of proteins.

• *Causes/contributory factors of Kwashiorkor*:
    i. Large family size.
   ii. Poor health of mother.
  iii Premature termination of breastfeeding.
   iv. Poor environmental condition.
    v. Delayed supplementary feeding.
   vi. Use of diluted cows milk to the infants or children.

• *Symptoms/effects*:
    i. Retarded growth
   ii. Oedema

  iii. Changes or alteration in pigmentation of skin and hair

  iv. Changes in texture of skin

   v. Enlargement of liver

  vi. Hypoalbuminaemia

 vii. GIT disturbances

viii. Psychic changes

  ix. Hypoglycaemia

   x. Stools containing much higher quantity of digested food.

     – *Other symptoms*:
- Macrocytic anaemia
- Normocytic anaemia
- Decreased BMR
- Falling body temperature
- Fall in plasma levels of triglycerides, cholesterol, lipo-protein.

- *Treatments for Kwashiorkor*:
  - i. Supply of diet rich in protein.
  - ii. First choice milk and egg should be given, both being rich in proteins.
  - iii. Soybeans are best known vegetarian source of first class as well as second class proteins.
  - iv. Food from nonvegetarian source like liver, meat, sea food.
  - v. In severe condition blood transfusions are required.
  - vi. The use of preventive measures are best ways for avoiding this disease.

2. Marasmus disease (S. 00, 04; W. 00, 04)

It is the protein deficiency disease commonly found in infants below 1 year of age.

- *Causes*:
  - i. It is mainly caused due to deficiency of protiens and carbo-hydrates with same other nutritional factors.
  - ii. Protein and energy deficiency disease of such type is also known as marasmic kawshiorkor.
  - iii. It is commonly found in people in absence of maintaining proper diet.
  - iv. Early stop breastfeeding.
- *Symptoms*:
  - i. Retarded growth

    ii. Complete loss of body fat
   iii. Weakness
   iv. Changes in texture of skin
    v. Alteration in pigmentation of skin and hair
   vi. GIT disturbances
  vii. Oedema.
- *Treatment*:
    i. Providing diet rich in calories
   ii. Providing protein diet
  iii. Other nutritional factors is best course in prevention and cure of the marasmus.

3. *Nutritional Oedema*

This is a disease caused by prolonged and significant protein deficiency commonly found in adults.
- *Symptoms*:
     i. Loss of body weight
    ii. Reduced subcutaneous fat
   iii. Anaemia
   iv. Much higher susceptibility to the infection
    v. General lethargy
   vi. Increase in frequency of watery stools
  vii. Inability to carry-out sustained work
 viii. Delay in healing of wounds
   ix. Inability to carry-out prolonged hard work
    x. Oedema
- *Treatments*:
    i. The diet consisting mainly of milk, milk products, eggs and soybean is given.
   ii. It is always better to adopt preventive action by regulating protein content of daily diet.

Q 13. Write a note on inborn errors of amino acid metabolism. Explain metabolic disorders of amino acid metabolism.

Abnormal Amino Acid Metabolism

1. Phenylketonuria
2. Alkaptonuria
3. Maple syrup urine disease
4. Hartnups disease

1. *Phenylketonuria (S. 04, 05, 07; W. 00, 02, 04, 06, 07)*

- This is a genetic disorder related to the phenylalanine metabolisms.

- Phenylalanine is a precursor for the biosynthesis of tyrosine.
- In this disorder, there is inherited deficiency of phenylalanine hydroxylase enzyme.
- This leads to accumulation of phenylalanine and it is excreted as phenylpyruvate. This conditions is called phenylketonuria.
- Due to deficiency to tyrosine, mental retardation is seen in young infants.

$$\text{Phenylalanine} + O_2 \xrightarrow[\text{Hydroxylase}]{\text{Phenylalanine}} \text{Tyrosine}$$

Symptoms:
- i. Retardation of mental growth in infants and children.
- ii. Deficiency of neurotransmitter serotonin leading to defect in myelin sheath of myelinated nerve fibres.
- iii. Disturbed synthesis of alanine.
- iv. Abnormal skin and hair.
- v. Excretion of various abnormal metabolites through the urine.

Treatment:
- i. Early diagnosis very shortly after birth
- ii. Restriction upon intake of phenylalanine.

2. *Alkaptonuria (W. 02, 04, 06, 07)*

- It is an inborn metabolic disorder of phenylalanine where there is an accumulation of homogentisic acid.
- This disorder is due to deficiency of enzyme homogentisate oxidase.
- As a result metabolism of homogentisic acid is blocked.
- Thus homogentisic acid accumulates in blood at high levels and so also it is excreted through the urine.
- Thus condition is seen to be present right from the birth and persist throughout the life of affected person.

$$\text{Homogentisic acid} \xrightarrow[\substack{\text{Homogentisate} \\ \text{oxidase}}]{O_2} \text{Maleyl acetoacetic acid}$$

Symptoms:
- i. Accumulation of homogentisic acid in blood and its excretion through the urine.
- ii. Dark black urine is excreted.
- iii. Accumulation of dark (blue black) pigment in tendons, cartilages, other connective tissues, skin of face, nails, etc.

    iv. Arthritis.

    v. Changes in heart valves due to accumulation of homogentisic acid.

3. *Maple Syrup Urine Disease (Urine Maple Syrup)* (S. 01, 04, 05, 07; W. 97)

- It is characterised by absence of enzyme responsible for oxidative decarboxylation of keto acids.
- Such keto acids are normally derived from branched chain amino acids like valine, lucine and isoleucine.
- It is an inborn metabolic disorder seen in the infants and resulting in blocking normal metabolism of keto acids and the amino acids.
- Final result is accumulation of keto acid derivatives of corresponding amino acid in the blood and some abnormal derivatives are excreted through urine.

Symptoms:

    i. Keto acid derivatives present in blood and their excretion through the urine.

    ii. Vomiting.

    iii. Lethargy (dullness).

    iv. Difficulty in speech in the infants.

    v. Apnoea (difficulty in breathing).

    vi. Convulsions.

    This disease is called maple syrup urine disease because the urine of affected person smells like maple syrup or burnt sugar.

4. *Hartnups Disease*

- It is inborn metabolic disorder of amino acid tryptophan.
- This disease is caused due to deficiency of enzyme 'tryptophan pyrroles' which results into accumulation of tryptophan and its derivatives indole acetic acid, indole pyruvic acid, in the blood.
- After this there is excretion of these acids in the urine.

Symptoms:

    i. Pellagra like dermatitis

    ii. Mental retardation

    iii. Urine with large amounts of indole acetic acid and indole pyruvic acid

    iv. The faeces containing large amount of tryptophan

    v. Deficiency of nicotinic acid.

4

Carbohydrates

Q 1. Define carbohydrates. Classify carbohydrates with examples. (S. 96, 98, 99, 00, 02, 03, 04, 07, 09; W. 97, 98, 99, 00, 02, 03, 05, 06, 07)

Carbohydrates

"Carbohydrates can be defined as organic compounds which are polyhydroxy aldehydes or polyhydroxy ketones or their derivative or substances which upon hydrolysis gives these derivatives."

Carbohydrates are also called as saccharides meaning sugar.

Classification of Carbohydrates

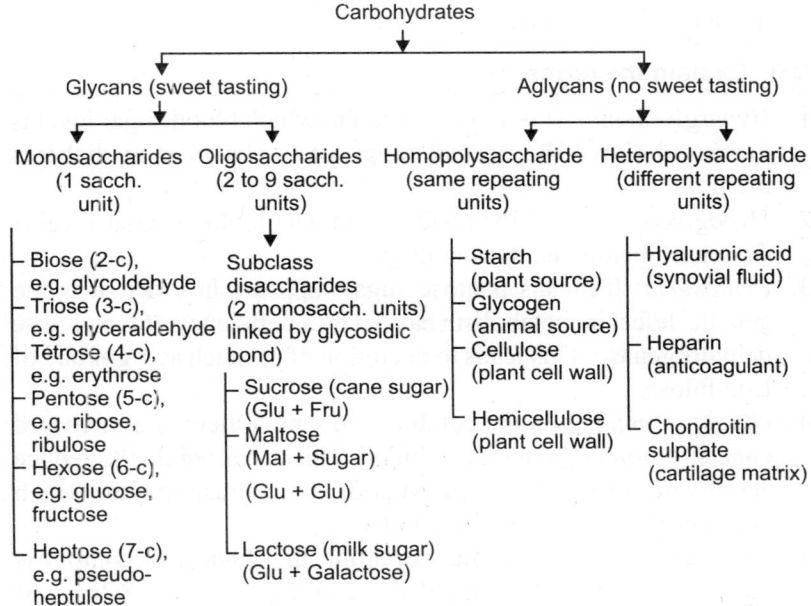

Q 2. Give the biological role/function/importance of carbohydrates. (S. 99; W. 96)

- Carbohydrates works as a main source of energy.
- Glucose is a readily available energy source.
- Glucose, fructose, galactose all the three are rich source of energy.
- Glycogen is reservoir of energy, where glycogen is stored in the liver and skeletal muscles.
- Carbohydrates are required as structural building blocks for synthesis of carbohydrates.
- Cerebrosides are special carbohydrates being provided to the nervous tissue.
- Cellulose and hemicellulose though do not posses energy value there function is to clean alimentary canal as they possess roughage value.
- Derivatives of glucose and galactose are required to synthesize special polysaccharides as heparin and chondroitins sulphate (part of structure of cartilage).
- Ribose is useful for nucleic acid synthesis.
- Galactose is necessary for forming lactose of milk of glycoproteins.
- Starches are important food reserve for the plant and food stuff for men and other animals.

Q 3. Explain the terms.

1. *Hyperglycaemia*: It is the condition in which blood sugar level is increased above the normal range. It is observed in diabetes mellitus.

2. *Hypoglycaemia*: It is the condition in which blood sugar level is decreased below the normal range.

3. *Pentosuria*: It means pentose sugars appears in urine. It is the genetic defect in metabolism caused by a deficiency of L-xylulose dehydrogenase. This leads to excretion of as much as 1 gm/day of L-xylulose.

4. *Galactosaemia*: It is the condition in which there is a increased concentration of galactose in blood. This is caused due to reduce activity of glucose-1-phosphate uridyl transferase enzyme which is essential for galactose metabolism.

5. *Polyuria*: It is an abnormal condition in which urine output is much higher than the normal urine output, i.e. 3 to 8 litres of urine per day.

Q 4. Draw the structures of following sugars. (S. 99, 00, 01, 02; W. 97, 00, 03, 04)

i. Glucose (S. 05, 06; W. 05)   ii. Fructose (S. 05, 06; W. 05, 07)

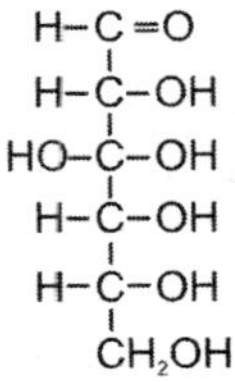

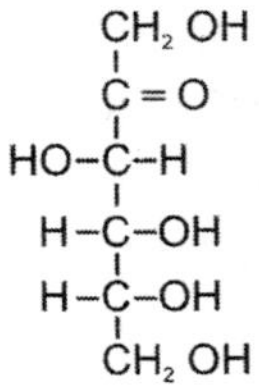

```
H-C=O                    CH₂OH
H-C-OH                   C=O
HO-C-OH                  HO-C-H
H-C-OH                   H-C-OH
H-C-OH                   H-C-OH
CH₂OH                    CH₂OH
```

iii. Sucrose (S. 96, 98, 02, 03, 06, 07, 08; W. 97, 01, 07)

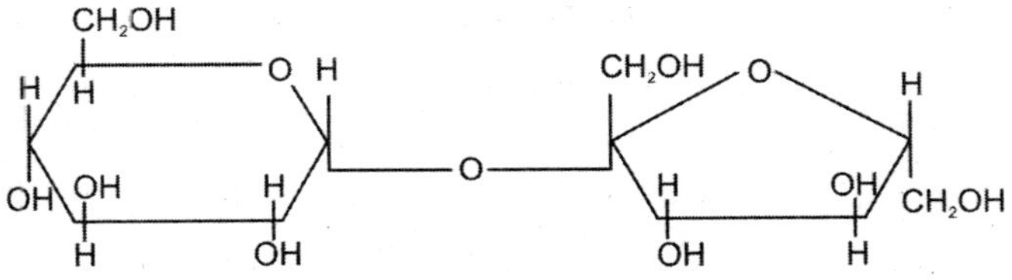

(Glucose)   (Fructose)

iv. Maltose (S. 98, 06, 07; W. 96, 97, 07)

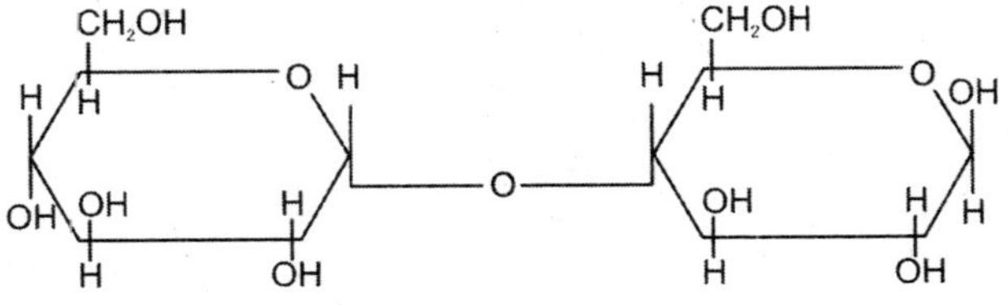

(Glucose)   (Glucose)

v. Lactose (S. 02, 06, 07, 08; W. 96, 99, 07)

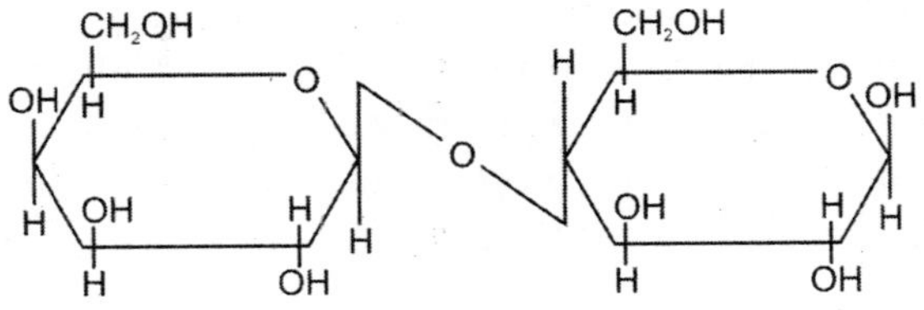

Q.5. Explain osazone test for carbohydrates (glucose)? (What is the action of phenylhydrazine on carbohydrates). (S. 03, 04, 05, 06, 07, 08, 09; W. 03, 06)

Osazone test is used to detect and distinguish the reducing sugar. When reducing sugar is treated with phenylhydrazine under boiling temperature and alkaline medium, there is a formation of osazone crystals. There crystals are water insoluble and yellow coloured. These are seen under microscope. The shape and arrangement of these crystals for the particular reducing sugar is different.

- *Reaction*:

1.
$$\begin{array}{l} \text{CHO} \\ | \\ \text{H}-\text{C}-\text{OH} \\ | \\ (\text{CHOH})_3 \\ | \\ \text{CH}_2\text{OH} \end{array} \quad \xrightarrow[\substack{\text{in alkaline medium} \\ \text{(boiling temperature)}}]{C_6H_5NH \cdot NH_2} \quad \begin{array}{l} \text{CH}=\text{N}\cdot\text{NH}\cdot\text{C}_6\text{H}_5 \\ | \\ \text{H}-\text{C}-\text{OH} \\ | \\ (\text{CHOH})_3 \quad + \text{H}_2\text{O} \\ | \\ \text{CH}_2\text{OH} \end{array}$$

D-glucose   Glucose phenylhydrazone

2.
$$\begin{array}{l} \text{CH}=\text{N}\cdot\text{NH}\cdot\text{C}_6\text{H}_5 \\ | \\ \text{H}-\text{C}-\text{OH} \\ | \\ (\text{CHOH})_3 \\ | \\ \text{CH}_2\text{OH} \end{array} \quad \xrightarrow[\substack{\text{in alkaline medium} \\ \text{(boiling temperature)}}]{C_6H_5NH \, NH_2} \quad \begin{array}{l} \text{CH}=\text{N}\cdot\text{NH}\cdot\text{C}_6\text{H}_5 \\ | \\ \text{C}=\text{O} \\ | \\ (\text{CHOH})_3 \quad + \text{C}_6\text{H}_5\text{NH}_2 + \text{NH}_3 \\ | \\ \text{CH}_2\text{OH} \quad \text{Aniline Ammonia} \end{array}$$

Glucose phenylhydrazone

3.
$$\begin{array}{l} \text{CH}=\text{N}\cdot\text{NH}\cdot\text{C}_6\text{H}_5 \\ | \\ \text{C}=\text{O} \\ | \\ (\text{CHOH})_3 \\ | \\ \text{CH}_2\text{OH} \end{array} \quad \xrightarrow[\substack{\text{in alkaline medium} \\ \text{(boiling temperature)}}]{C_6H_5NH \cdot NH_2} \quad \begin{array}{l} \text{CH}=\text{N}\cdot\text{NH}\cdot\text{C}_6\text{H}_5 \\ | \\ \text{C}=\text{N}\cdot\text{NH}\cdot\text{C}_6\text{H}_5 \\ | \\ (\text{CHOH})_3 \quad + \text{H}_2\text{O} \\ | \\ \text{CH}_2\text{OH} \end{array}$$

Glucosazone

- *Mechanism of osazone formation:*
    i. When reducing sugar is treated with phenylhydrazine, it gives the reaction product phenylhydrazine.
    ii. The two molecules are heated again with phenylhydrazine, it gives rise to products like aniline, ammonia, and glucosazone.
    iii. In actual mechanism three molecules of phenylhydrazine hydrochloride react with one molecule of reducing sugar to produce one osazone crystal of respective reducing sugar, e.g. glucose, fructose, galactose.

- Osazones of different reducing sugars are as follows:
    - i. Glucose   — Glucosazones

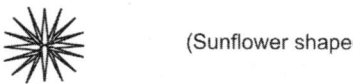

(Needle shaped)

    - ii. Lactose   — Lactosazones

(Balls of prickles like shape)

    - iii. Maltosazones — Maltose

(Sunflower shaped)

- *Significance of osazone test:*
    - i. Osazone test helps to differentiate reducing sugars from non-reducing sugars like starch, dextrin, sucrose.
    - ii. Osazone test also helps to differentiate particular type of reducing sugar differentiate it from other types reducing sugars.
    - iii. Osazone test is used to identify and confirm reducing sugars, e.g. glucose, fructose, galactose, maltose, lactose (disaccharides).

Q 6. Give the biological role and functions of glucose.

Functions of Glucose

1. Glucose is very easily available and ready to use source of energy for all living cells.
2. Glucose is best suitable transport form of sugar due to its high water solubility.
3. Mainly riped fruits are sweet tasting because they contains glucose.
4. One molecule of glucose after complete oxidation provides 673 kg cal energy, equivalent to 38 ATPs. So glucose is rich and ideal source of energy.
5. Different derivatives of glucose are important intermediates of carbohydrate metabolism.
6. Glucosamine is another important amino sugar of glucose which is structural part of some antibiotics as like erythromycin, streptomycin.
7. Glucose is an important structural part of complex polysaccharides as starch, cellulose, hemicellulose and the glycogen.

8. Glucose is structural unit of biologically important disaccharide as maltose, sucrose and lactose.
9. Glucose can be converted into the water insoluble form called glycogen via glycogenesis process.

Q 7. Write a note on oxidation of glucose. (W. 03)

Sugar on oxidation gives acid. The oxidation product depend upon oxidising agent used in the reaction.

Glucose is oxidised to different products with the help of different oxidising agents.

i. Oxidation of 1st carbon

$$
\begin{array}{ccc}
\text{CHO} & & \text{COOH} \\
| & & | \\
\text{(CHOH)}_4 & \xrightarrow[\text{Na-hypo-iodite}]{\text{Br}_2 \text{ H}_2\text{O}} & \text{(CHOH)}_4 \\
| & & | \\
\text{CH}_2\text{OH} & & \text{CH}_2\text{OH} \\
\text{D-glucose} & & \text{(Aldonic acid)} \\
& & \text{Gluconic acid}
\end{array}
$$

ii. Oxidation of 6th carbon

$$
\begin{array}{ccc}
\text{CHO} & & \text{CHO} \\
| & & | \\
\text{(CHOH)}_4 & \xrightarrow[\text{O}_2]{\text{Pt}} & \text{(CHOH)}_4 \\
| & & | \\
\text{CH}_2\text{OH} & & \text{COOH} \\
\text{D-glucose} & & \text{(Uronic acid)} \\
& & \text{Glucoronic acid}
\end{array}
$$

iii. Oxidation of 1st and 6th carbon

$$
\begin{array}{ccc}
\text{CHO} & & \text{COOH} \\
| & & | \\
\text{(CHOH)}_4 & \xrightarrow{\text{Conc. HNO}_3} & \text{(CHOH)}_4 \\
| & & | \\
\text{CH}_2\text{OH} & & \text{COOH} \\
\text{D-glucose} & & \text{(Saccharic acid)} \\
& & \text{Glucosaccharic acid}
\end{array}
$$

i. *Aldonic acid formation*: When glucose is treated with mild oxidising agents like bromine water and Na-hypoiodite, the product generated is aldonic acid. Here the 1st carbon from CHO group of glucose is oxidised and replaced by carboxyl (–COOH) group. The product formed is generally called aldonic acid while for glucose it is called gluconic acid.

ii. *Uronic acid formation (oxidation at 6th carbon)*: When glucose is treated with better strong oxidising agent as platinum and molecular O_2, there is an oxidation of 6th carbon in CH_2OH group of glucose. Hence oxidation replaces the CH_2OH by –COOH (carboxyl group). In general product formed is called uronic acid while for glucose it is called glucoronic acid.

iii. *Saccharic acid formation (oxidation of both 1st and 6th carbon)*: Here the glucose is treated with very strong oxidising agent as concentration HNO_3, where both 1st and 6th carbons are oxidised and replaced by carboxyl (–COOH) group. The product formed in general is called saccharic acid. While for glucose it is called glucosaccharic acid.

Q 8. What are reducing sugar? Write a note on reducing sugars. (S. 96, 97, 01, 06, 09)

Reducing Sugars

There are the sugars possessing free aldehyde or ketone group in their structure and possess an ability to reduce certain heavy metal ions, e.g. glucose, fructose, galactose, lactose, maltose presence of free aromatic carbon atom possess an ability to reduce certain heavy metal ions. This is called the reducing property of reducing sugars. In this reaction the precipitation of specific colour is obtained, which can indicate roughly the amount of reducing sugar present, e.g. copper ions present in Fehling and Benedicts reagent can be reduced in alkaline medium at high temperature to form cuprous oxide by reducing ability of monosaccharides. The reactions can be operated as follows:

i. $CuSO_4 \longrightarrow Cu^{++} + SO_4^{--}$

ii. Reducing sugar $\xrightarrow[\substack{\text{Alkaline medium and} \\ \text{high temperature}}]{Na_2CO_3}$ Enediol form of reducing sugar

iii. Cu^{++} enediol form of sugar $\longrightarrow Cu^{++} +$ Mixture of sugar acids.

iv. $Cu^{++} + OH^-$ from sugar acids $\longrightarrow CuOH$.

v. $2\,CuOH \longrightarrow Cu_2O + H_2O$

This particular mechanism of reaction of metallic ion forms common basis to detect all reducing sugar.

The colour of precipitation obtained in observation, tell about approximate amount of reducing sugar present in corresponding sugar solution.

Colour precipitation	Approximate % of reducing sugar
Greenish colour precipitation	0.5 (+)
Green colour precipitation	0.5 to 1 (++)
Yellow colour precipitation	1 to 1.5 (+++)
Yellow to orange colour precipitation	1.5 to 2 (++++)
Dark brick red colour precipitation	More than 2 (+++++)

Significance

Benedicts qualitative test posses a diagnostic value, where this test is used to detect roughly the amount of reducing sugar, if present in urine sample, in detectable amount. The abnormal pathological condition indicating presence of reducing sugar in the urine, in the detectable amount is called glycosuria. Very typically glycosuria is prominent of disease diabetes mellitus.

Q 9. Write a note on "diabetes mellitus". (S. 99, 01; W. 99, 00, 04)

Diabetes mellitus is a condition caused due to raised glucose concentration in the blood due to deficiency of insulin.

Types of Diabetes Mellitus

   i. Juvenile-onset type of diabetes mellitus (10 to 12 years).

   ii. Maturing onset type of diabetes mellitus (middle or/later ages).

Symptoms/Characteristics of Diabetes Mellitus

- Hyperglycaemia
- Glycosuria
- Weakness/tiredness
- Loss of body weight
- Intense thirst (polydypsia)
- Dehydration
- Breathlessness

- Polyuria
- Reduced visual activity
- Epigastric pain and vomiting
- Pains in legs
- Infection of skin, lung and urinary tract
- Dry skin, cracked lips
- Rapid pulse, BP is low.

Causes of Diabetes Mellitus

- Genetic factors
- Obesity
- Dietary intake of sugar in excess
- Increased rate of glucose absorption from intestine
- Decreased level of insulin.

Treatment

- Use of oral antidiabetic agents and insulin
- High protein and low carbohydrate and fat diet are advisable.

Q 10. What is glycosuria? (S. 97, 01, 04; W. 96)

Glycosuria

The condition in which an abnormal quantities of glucose is excreted in the urine is called glycosuria. Glycosuria can be classified as follows:

   i. *Alimentary glycosuria*: Glucose may appear in urine temporarily due to high intake of carbohydrate, without any defect in blood glucose regulatory mechanism. This is known as alimentary glycosuria.

   ii. *Renal glycosuria*: In this case there are defects in tubular mechanism that leads to glucose excretion in urine.

   iii. *Diabetic glycosuria*: This type of glycosuria occur in diabetes mellitus due to hyperglycemia resulting from insulin deficiency.

Q 11. Write a note on 'mutarotation' of carbohydrates. (S. 96, 97, 03; W. 96, 02, 04, 05, 06, 07)

Mutarotation

"The change in specific rotation of plane polarized light by solution of optically active substance but without any change in other properties of that compound, is known as mutarotation."

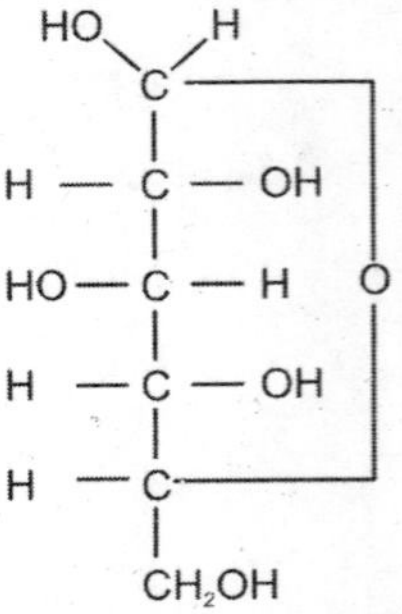

α -form of D-glucose

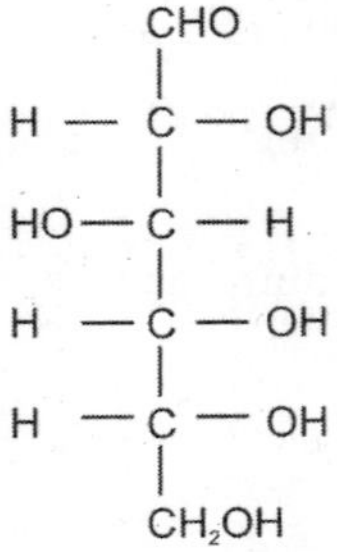

D-glucose

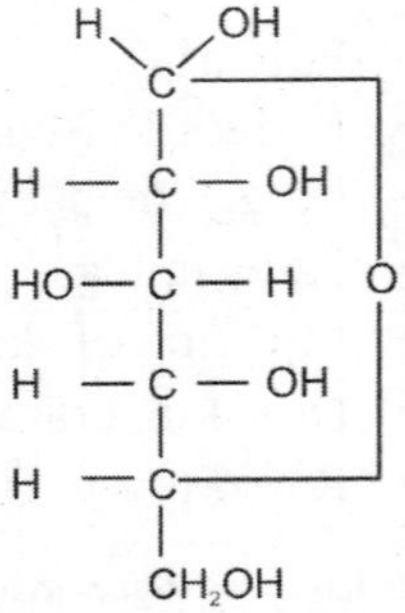

β-from of D-glucose

When a carbohydrate compound carries asymmetric carbon, it show optical activity, i.e. ability to rotate plane polarized light, e.g. glucose as hexose sugar exist in α and β-forms shown above.

When glucose is dissolved in water, optical rotation of solution gradually changes to attend the equilibrium. This change in optical rotation as shown below is called mutarotation.

α- D-glucose (36%) ⇌ Glucose ⇌ β-D-glucose (63%)
(+ 112.2°)   (+ 52.5°)   (+ 19°)

Equilibrium mixture of α and β-forms of
D-glucose and with open chain form of glucose

Main reason of mutarotation is formation of cyclic or ring compound from the open chain form of D-glucose. α and β-forms of D-glucose differ from each other only with respect to rotation. Under such condition α-form shows optical activity + 112.2° and β-form shows optical activity + 19°. Initially in aqueous solution α and β-forms are in different properties as 36% and 63% respectively. Later on in the mixture, equilibrium status of α and β-forms is achieved. Initially much high percentage of β-form is present because of its stable configuration relative to α-form. Finally when equilibriums mixture of α and β-form is achieved, the optical rotation changes and stabilizes to + 52.5°.

In the biological system, i.e. living cells, such mutarotation is carried out by activity of enzyme called *mutarotase*.

Q 12. Write a note on cellulose (location and importance).

Cellulose is a hormopolysaccharide. Cellulose is a linear unbranched long chain polymer of D-glucose unit linked by β-1,4-glycoside bond.

Location of Cellulose

  i. It occurs in plant tissues but totally absent in the animal tissue.
 ii. Actually in plant tissues cellulose is present as a structural part of cell wall.
iii. Cellulose is distinctly present in the wood and fibrous tissues in one plant body.

Importance of Cellulose

  i. For human body cellulose fibres possess roughage value, i.e. they act as a cleansing plug.
 ii. Cotton and filter papers are the examples of true cellulose and are of great commercial value.
iii. Fibres of jute and hemp are of commercial use in cordage industries.

Q 13. Differentiate between starch and glycogen.

Starch	Glycogen
1. Storage form of carbohydrate for the plant.	1. Storage form of carbohydrate for the animals.
2. It is insoluble in water.	2. It is better soluble in water.
3. It shows less branched structure.	3. It shows highly branched structure.
4. Branching repeat after every 25 to 30 glucose units.	4. Branching repeat after every 8 to 10 glucose units.
5. For iodine test it gives dark blue violet colour.	5. For iodine test it gives dark pinkish red to brown colour.
6. It is digested by action of different digestive enzymes which come from salivary glands, pancreas and intestinal mucosa.	6. Metabolism of glycogen occurs by special mechanism called Cori cycle, promoted by glycogenolysis and enzyme LDH.
7. The location for breakdown of starch is cavity within alimentary canal.	7. The location for breakdown of glycogen are mainly skeletal muscle and liver.
8. It is very common part of the human diet.	8. It is very less frequently part of the human diet.

Q 14. Explain enediol formation/enolisation of carbohydrate. Explain action of dilute alkali on sugars (glucose).

When monosaccharide is heated with dilute alkali like KOH or NaOH solution, there is formation of enediol form of the monosaccharide.

Both aldose and ketose (–C=O) type of sugars gives this test positive. The enediol form carries C=C in C-1 and C-2 of the concerned monosaccharide. Such process of enediol formation is called enolisation.

$$
\begin{array}{ccc}
\text{CHO} & & \text{HO–C–H} \\
\text{H–C–OH} & & \text{C–OH} \\
\text{HO–C–H} & \xrightarrow[\substack{\text{Dilute alkali} \\ \text{(KOH/NaOH solution)}}]{\text{Enolisation}} & \text{HO–C–H} \\
\text{H–C–OH} & & \text{H–C–OH} \\
\text{H–C–OH} & & \text{H–C–OH} \\
\text{CH}_2\text{OH} & & \text{CH}_2\text{OH}
\end{array}
$$

(1,2-enediol form of glucose)

Q 15. Explain various qualitative chemical tests for identification of carbohydrates.

Qualitative Tests for Carbohydrates

1. Benedict test ⎫
2. Felhings test ⎬ Test for reducing sugars
3. Barfoeds test ⎭
4. Molish test
5. Mucic acid test
6. Seliwanoffs test
7. Tollens mirror test
8. Iodine test
9. Osazone test

1. *Benedict test (S. 99, 04; W. 99, 02)*: This test is positive for all reducing sugars. Benedicts reagent contains cupric ions (cupric sulphate) in alkaline medium and different chelating agents to keep the cupric ions in solution. When sugar is heated with Benedict reagent the **cupric ions** are reduced to **cuprous ions** which gives brick red or yellow precipitate depending upon the concentration of sugar.

The brick red precipitate indicates the presence of 'monosaccharides'.

2. *Felhings test (S. 99, 02)*: Felhings solution is a cupric tartrate alkaline solution. This test is positive to all reducing sugars.

The Felhings solution is composed of copper sulphate, sodium potassium tartarte and potassium hydroxide.

Carbohydrates with free aldehyde and ketone groups having an ability to reduce and copper sulphate to cuprous oxide forming a yellow or brownish red coloured precipitate.

Test: Boil sugar solution and Felhing solution for two minutes gives formation of brick red precipitate which indicates the reducing sugar.

3. *Barfoeds test*: This test is positive for monosaccharides. This reagent contains cupric acetate and dilute acetic acid. The monosaccharides when heated with Barfoeds reagent, Cu^{++} is reduced to Cu^+ where later on Cu^+ is precipitated to cuprous oxide forming red or brick red precipitate.

   The reducing disaccharides reduce Barfoeds reagent very slowly as compared to monosaccharides.

   • *Significance*: This test is used to distinguish reducing monosaccharides from reducing disaccharides.

4. *Seliwanoffs test*: It is the typical test for ketose type of sugar that produces a cherry-red or reddish brown colour on boiling for half minute with Seliwanoffs reagent containing resorcinol in HCl. The same colour is produced on prolonged boiling of an aldose solution with Seliwanoffs reagent.

5. *Iodine test*: Iodine in aqueous solution reacts with different types of carbohydrates to give different kinds of specific coloured compounds, e.g.

   Starch   + I_2 ⎯⎯⎯→ Blue violet

   Dextrin + I_2 ⎯⎯⎯→ Pink

   Glycogen + I_2 ⎯⎯⎯→ Brown

   Amylose + I_2 ⎯⎯⎯→ Deep blue

6. *Molish test* (*S. 99, 02; W. 99, 02*): It is the general test for identification of carbohydrates.

   • *Principle*: In this test carbohydrate reacts with strong mineral acids like Conc. H_2SO_4 to produce furfural compound. The furfural compound in 2nd step interact with α-naphthol to produce blue violet colour conjugate because of alcoholic α-naphthol and strong mineral acid are not miscible with each other.

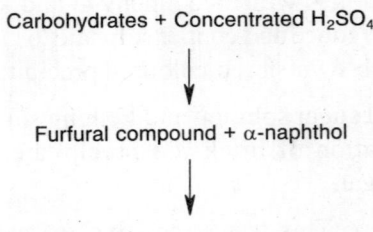

Carbohydrates + Concentrated H_2SO_4

↓

Furfural compound + α-naphthol

↓

Blue violet ring at the junction

- *Observation*: The violet coloured compound forms the ring at the junction of two immiscible liquids.
- *Significance:*
    i. This test is commonly used for identification of all carbohydrates.
    ii. This test distinguishes the carbohydrates from all other organic compounds.

7. *Mucic acid test*: It is the typical test give positive by galactose as hexose sugar. In actual test galactose is treated with strong oxidizing agents as concentrated HNO_3. In this reaction both carbon 1 and 6 get oxidised and replaced by carboxyl (–COOH) group. The end product obtained is called galactosaccharic acid or mucic acid.

    This compound occurs as a broken glass and so it is very typical confirmatory test for galactose.

    Actually mucic acid forms colourless, water insoluble crystals of broken glass type seen.

    Reaction can be represented as:

```
        CHO                           COOH
     H–C–OH                        H–C–OH
    HO–C–H      Conc. HNO₃        HO–C–H
    HO–C–H      ──────────→       H–C–H
     H–C–OH                        H–C–OH
      CH₂OH                         CH₂OH   Mucic acid
     Galactose                  (Broken glass crystals)
```

8. *Tollen's mirror test/silver mirror test*: Reducing disaccharides commonly gives positive test for Tollen's reagent.

    The sugar is heated with ammoniacal silver nitrate solution. If the sugar has a free aldehyde or ketone group, it changes to enediol which then reduces Ag^{++} to metallic silver precipitating it in the form of a **shining mirror**.

- *Test*: Sugar is heated with Tollen's reagent, a silver mirror is obtained inside the wall of vessel indicates the presence of aldoses.

Q 16. What are anomers and epimers. (S. 97; W. 04)

Anomers

Two isomeric forms of D ($\neq$) glucose, i.e. $\alpha - (+)$ glucose and $\beta -$ D (+) glucose are diastereomers differing in configuration about C–1. Such a pair of diastereomers are called anomers.

Epimers

A pair of diastereomeric aldoses that differ only in configuration about C–2 are called epimers.

5

Lipids

Q 1. What are lipids? Classify with suitable examples. (S. 98, 99, 00, 02, 04, 05, 09; W. 96, 99, 00, 07)

Lipids

"Lipids are heterogenous group of organic compounds related to fatty acids which are insoluble in water and soluble in organic solvents like ether, chloroform and benzene."

Classification of Lipids

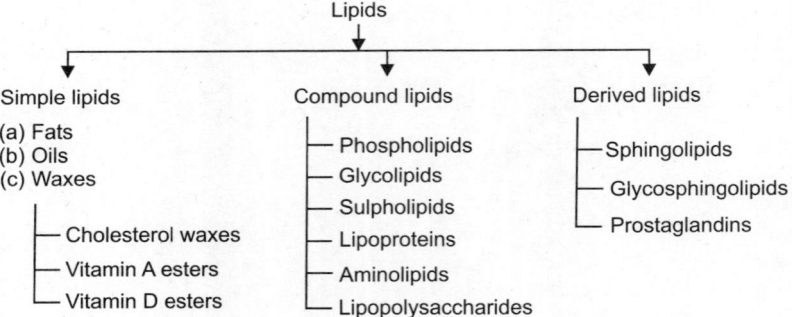

Q 2. Give biological functions or physiological role of lipids. (S. 96, 98, 99, 00, 02, 03, 05, 06; W. 96, 97, 99, 01, 02, 04, 08)

1. Lipids, fats and oils are important constituents of daily diet of human beings.
2. Lipids acts as an efficient source of energy when stored in adipose tissues.
3. Lipids serves as an insulating materials in the subcutaneous tissue and certain organs.
4. Lipids provides essential fatty acids which are not synthesized by human body.

5. Lipids are the carriers of fat soluble vitamins.
6. Lipids helps to maintain functions of cells of the body, e.g. lipoproteins.
7. Lipids provide building blocks for different high molecular weight substances, e.g. cholesterol, hormones.
8. Lipids produce metabolites which are used in the interconversion of substances.
9. Fats serves as a fuel molecule.
10. In myelinated nerve fibre, axon is covered with myelin sheath which is fatty sheath.
11. Derived lipids like steroids are most important building blocks for steroid hormones, e.g. sex hormones, adrenal hormones.
12. Fats provides mechanical support and so protect vitally important organs against mechanical injuries, e.g. heart, major blood vessels, kidneys, spinal cord are supported by fats.

Q 3. What are essential fatty acids? Give examples. (S. 96, 04, 07; W. 01, 02, 03, 05, 07)

Essential Fatty Acids

"The unsaturated fatty acids which are not synthesized in the body and are required for the growth of body are called as essential fatty acids."

They are supplied from diet.

Examples
  i. Linoleic acid
 ii. Linolenic acid
iii. Arachidonic acid.

Deficiency of Essential Fatty Acids

1. Dry and scaly skin
2. Loss of hairs
3. Poor and delayed wound healing
4. Slow growth
5. Retarded growth
6. Increased BMR.

Importance/Functions of Essential Fatty Acids

1. In high concentration along with lipids constitutes the structural elements of tissues.

2. They helps in synthesis of prostaglandins.
3. They prolongs clotting time.
4. They retard arthrosclerosis.
5. They cure skin lesions.
6. The deficiencies of these acids in the diet of babies causes eczema.

Q 4. What are "saturated and unsaturated fatty acids"? Give examples.

Saturated Fatty Acids

"The fatty acids which contains straight chain saturated hydrocarbon are called as saturated fatty acids."

$$\left[\begin{array}{c} | \; | \\ -C-C- \\ | \; | \end{array} \right]$$

For example: Palmitic acid, stearic acid, caproic acid.

Unsaturated Fatty Acids ($-C{=}C-$)

"The fatty acids which have one or more double bonds in their molecules are called as unsaturated fatty acids," e.g. oleic acid, linolenic acid, arachidonic acid.

Q 5. Define 'fats', 'oils' and 'waxes'. (S. 08; W. 07)

Fats

Fats are the esters of fatty acids with glycerol and are solid at ordinary temperature (20°C).

Oils

Oils are the esters of fatty acids with glycerol and are liquid at room temperature (20°C).

Waxes Fats

Waxes are the esters of fatty acids with higher alcohol.

Q 6. Write a note on 'rancidity of oils and fats'/'rancidification'. (S. 96, 97, 98, 03, 08; W. 96, 97, 99, 03, 05, 07)

Rancidification

"When fat and oils are exposed to light, air, heat, moisture for a longer time, develops disagreeable and objectionable odour. Such oil or fat is said to be rancid. This phenomenon is called as rancidification."

- The bad and objectionable odour is because of liberation of volatile fatty acids like butyric acid, caproic acid, and caprylic acid.
- Oils and fats on long exposure to air turns rancid and develops disagreeable odour.
- The rancid oils or fats shows acidic reactions. This is due to partial decomposition of glyceride resulting into more amount of free acid.
- Rancid oils shows high acid values.
- Rancidity is of two types:
  a. *Hydrolytic rancidity*: Some oils and fats undergo hydrolysis and produce bad odour is called hydrolytic rancidity.
  b. *Oxidative rancidity*: It is the rancidity caused due to oxidation of double bonds in fats and oils.
- Addition of some substances called as antioxidants can prevent the rancidity of fats and oils.
- Vitamin E, ascorbic acid and some derivatives of phenol are some examples of antioxidants.
- Addition of antioxidants can prolong or increase the shelf-life of food containing fats and oils.
- There are some substances called as pro-oxidants which in fact promote and carry out rapidly the rancidity of fats and oils. Some examples of pro-oxidants are copper, lead, nickel, etc.

Q 7. Give the physical properties of fats and oils. (W. 03)

1. Fats are solid at room temperature while oils are liquid at room temperature.
2. These are insoluble in water but soluble in organic solvents like ether, benzene, chloroform, etc.
3. Fats are colourless, odourless and tasteless.
4. Fats are neutral in action and so do not show any change in litmus paper colour upon reaction.
5. Fats possess comparatively low melting point.
6. Fats and oils spread uniformly over the surface of water by mono-layer formation.
   - *Chemical properties*:
     1. Hydrolysis
     2. Acrolein formation
     3. Halogenation
     4. Oxidation

5. Rancidity
6. Saponification
7. Hydrogenation.

Q 8. Write a note on 'acrolein formation'.

$$
\begin{array}{c}
\underset{\text{Glycerol}}{
\begin{array}{l}
CH_2OH \\
| \\
CH-OH \\
| \\
CH_2OH
\end{array}
}
\quad
\underset{KHSO_4}{\xrightarrow{\substack{\text{Heating in} \\ \text{presence of}}}}
\quad
\underset{\text{(Acrolein)}}{
\begin{array}{l}
CHO \\
| \\
CH \\
|| \\
CH_2
\end{array}
}
\; + H_2O
\end{array}
$$

When glycerol is heated with strong dehydrating agent as potassium bisulphate ($KHSO_4$). The product formed in called 'acrolein'. This product the acrolein posses characteristic strong irritating disagreeable or bad smell. Infect acrolein compound is identified on the basis of its particular smell only.

Acrolein formation reaction occurs in both cases where glycerol is either free or glycerol in esterified form in fats and oils as triglycerides. As $KHSO_4$ is strong dehydrating agent, this reaction also form water molecule.

By any reason if these occurs acrolein formation, for any fat or oil, then it becomes unsuitable for any use.

Q 9. Write a note on 'saponification./What are soaps? How are they synthesized?/Explain alkaline hydrolysis of fat and oil?

Saponification (Alkaline Hydrolysis of Fat or Oil) (S. 01, 02; W. 00, 07)

The hydrolysis of fat or oil by alkali gives the products like glycerol and alkali salts of fatty acids, i.e. soaps. This process is said to be saponification.

Generally the sodium and potassium salts of fatty acids are called as soaps.

$$
\underset{\text{(Triglycerides)}}{
\begin{array}{l}
CH_2-COOR \\
| \\
CH-COOR \\
| \\
CH_2-COOR
\end{array}
}
\underset{\text{(Alkali)}}{+\; 3\,NaOH}
\longrightarrow
\underset{\text{(Glycerol)}}{
\begin{array}{l}
CH_2OH \\
| \\
CH-OH \\
| \\
CH_2OH
\end{array}
}
\underset{\text{(Soaps)}}{+\; 3\,R-COONa}
$$

When soap is dissolved in water it forms an emulsion to produce soaps micelle which are stable arrangements of fat droplets. For each droplet polar heads are directed outwards and nonpolar tails are directed inwards, i.e. hidden inside micelle.

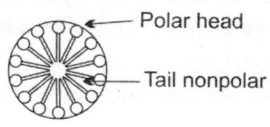

Soap micelle

The soap or the foam thus formed is not always stable. The stabilisation of soap depends upon formation of stable fat droplets or stable fat globules.

Soap can be stabilized by addition of stabilizing agents such as bile salts.

Q 10. Enlist various chemical constants for fat and oils/parameters used to study fats and oils (analysis of fats and oils) (IP standards for oils and fats).

1. Saponification number/sap value/soap value
2. Iodine value/number
3. Acetyl number/value
4. Acid number/value
5. Reicherts-Meissel number
6. Polenske number.

Q 11. Define and give significance of the following:

1. Saponification Number (Sap Value) (Soap Value) (S. 01, 02, 06, 09; W. 00, 03, 05, 07)

"It is defined as the number of milligrams of KOH or NaOH required to saponify 1 gm of oil or fat."

Saponification number is determined by saponification and titration of excess of alkali with fat or oil, e.g.

Fat or oil	Sap value
i. Butter fat	210–230 milligrams
ii. Human fat	195–200 milligrams
iii. Olive oil	185–195 milligrams
iv. Linseed oil	188–195 milligrams

Significance/Importance

   i. It tells about the content of free or bound fatty acids in a given fat or oil.

ii. It tells about the alkali required for conversion of fat into soap.

iii. It indicates the composition of oil or fat.

iv. It gives an estimate of nonfatty impurities in fat or oil.

v. A higher saponification number shows a high percentage of short chain acids in glycerides.

vi. It gives an idea about low molecular weight, if sap value is high.

2. Iodine Number (Iodine Value) (S. 99, 00, 01, 02, 06; W. 98, 00, 03, 04, 05, 07)

It is defined as number of grams of iodine absorbed by 100 gm of fat or oil.

- The unsaturation in a fat or oil is expressed in terms of iodine value.
- In actual reaction iodine is added to C=C of unsaturated fatty acids present in fat or oil. So unsaturation is removed, i.e. C=C. The halogenation reaction occurs as below:

$$R-CH=CH-COOH + I_2 \longrightarrow R-\overset{\overset{\displaystyle H}{|}}{\underset{|}{C}}-\overset{\overset{\displaystyle H}{|}}{\underset{|}{C}}-COOH$$

(Fatty acid present in oil or fat)

Iodine Value of Some Fats/Oils

i. Butter fat   26 to 28 gm

ii. Human fat   65 to 70 gm

Significance/Importance

i. It shows degree of unsaturation in fat or oil

ii. It helps in characterizing fat and oil

iii. It helps in finding out their suitability as a soap material.

3. Acid Number (Acid Value) (S. 98, 04, 06; W. 98, 01, 03, 04, 07)

It is defined as number of milligrams of KOH required to neutralize 1 gm of fat or oil.

Significance

i. It gives an idea about rancidity of oil or fat.

ii. It represents amount of free fatty acids in it.

iii. It helps to judge the quality of a given fat or oil, i.e. higher the acid value more is the rancidity.

4. Acetyl Number (Acetyl Value) (S. 98, 02, 04, 06, 07, 08, 09; W. 03)

It is defined as the number of milligram of KOH required for the neutralization of acetic acid obtained by saponification of 1 gm of an acetylated fat or oil.

Significance

By determining acetyl number the hydroxyl group present in fats or oil can be determined.

5. Reichert-Meissel Number (S. 07, 08; W. 01, 03, 06)

It is defined as the number of millilitres of 0.1 N KOH required to neutralise the soluble volatile fatty acids derived from 5 gm of fat or oil.

Significance

i. It helps to determine the amount of volatile fatty acids present in given fat or oil.

ii. This value is used to detect adulteration in fat or oil.

6. Polenske Number (S. 06; W. 01)

It is the number of millilitres of 0.1 N KOH required to neutralise the insoluble fatty acids from 5 gm of fat or oil.

Q 12. Enlist abnormalities in lipid metabolism. (S. 09)

Name the disease occurred due to disorders of lipid metabolism.
1. Obesity
2. Gauchers disease
3. Niemann-Picks disease
4. Hyperlipoproteinaemia
5. Hypolipoproteinaemia
6. Fabrys disease
7. Tay-Sachs disease.

Q 13. Explain the terms.

a. Obesity

Excessive deposition of fats in the depots with decreased mobility causes obesity. Obesity is caused due to ingestion of more food than necessary to meet the needs of the body.

Hypothyroidism, hyperinsulinism are other causes of obesity.

b. Gauchers Disease (S. 01)

- This is the disease associated with abnormal lipid metabolism.
- In this term there is an imbalance in both the synthesis and breakdown of cerebrosides.
- Thus cerebrosides are increased in the brain, liver and spleen.

Symptoms

    i. Enlargement of liver and spleen
   ii. Bone erosion
  iii. Mental retardation.

c. Niemann-Picks Disease (S. 01; W. 05)

- In this disease sphingomyelin accumulates in liver, spleen, bone marrow, lungs and lymph nodes.
- The abnormalities is an imbalance both synthesis and breakdown of the sphingomyelin.

Symptoms

    i. Enlargement of liver and spleen
   ii. Mental retardation
  iii. Red spot on retina.

d. Tay-Sachs Disease

This disease is characterized by abnormal accumulation of glycerides in the brain. The child does not usually survive beyond 2 to 4 years.

Symptoms

    i. Retarded development
   ii. Paralysis
  iii. Dementia
  iv. Blindness.

Q 14. Write a note on 'cholesterol'. (S. 06, 07, 09; W. 08)

Cholesterol

- Cholesterol is most important monohydric or steroid alcohol.
- Cholesterol makes structural part of biomembranes.
- Cholesterol is mainly synthesized in the liver. The rate of biosynthesis depends upon the fat content of the daily diet.
- Cholesterol is abundantly found in animal tissues.

- In conjugation with phospholipids it is found in the membrane.
- Cholesterol is precursor for bile salts, sex hormones, corticosteroids and vitamin D.

Structure of Cholesterol

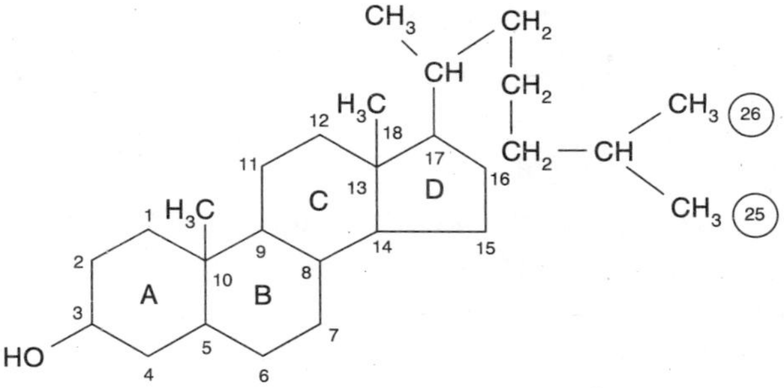

Functions/Importance of Cholesterol

   i. It forms a structural part of all biomembranes.

  ii. It acts as a precursors for biosynthesis of bile salts such as sodium glycocholate and sodium taurocholate.

 iii. It plays important role in biosynthesis of corticosteroid hormone such as glucocorticoids and mineralocorticoids. These two hormones together functions to relieve physical strain and mental stress.

 iv. It is required for the biosynthesis of male and female sex hormone or prostaglandins.

  v. Cholesterol is also the chief constituent of gallstones.

Abnormal Metabolism Related with Cholesterol

   i. Hypercholesterolaemia

  ii. Arteriosclerosis.

Colour Tests for Cholesterol **(S. 97, 02, 03, 06, 07; W. 98)**

   i. *Libermann Burchard reaction*: A chloroform solution of sterol when treated with acetic anhydride and sulphuric acid gives a green colour. This reaction is the basis of colorimetric estimation of blood cholesterol.

  ii. *Salkewski test*: When choroform solution of the sterol is treated with an equal volume of concentrated sulphuric acid it gives red to purple colour.

Q 15. Explain the role of lipids in biological membranes. (S. 98, 01; W. 02, 04, 05)

- The major component of biological membrane is phospholipid.
- Phospholipid has two long chains of hydrocarbon of fatty acids.

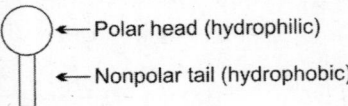

←— Polar head (hydrophilic)

←— Nonpolar tail (hydrophobic)

A Molecule of Phospholipid

- When phospholipids are added to aqueous medium they form micelles, monolayer and bilayer, depending on the concentration of phospholipid.

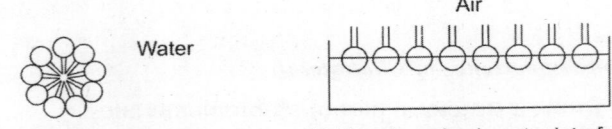

Water

Air

(a) Micelles in water   (b) Monolayer in air-water interface

- The hydrophilic and hydrophobic interaction of phospholipids are forming bilayer in water. Hydrophobic tails are hidden from aqueous environment and form an internal hydrophobic phase whereas the hydrophilic heads are exposed on the surface.
- Biomembranes are made up of phospholipids, lipoproteins, glycoproteins and proteins.

Fluid Mosaic Model of Biomembrane

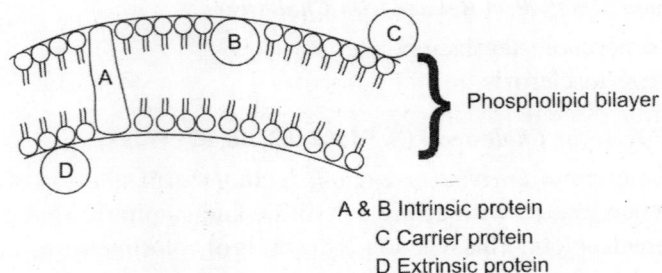

Phospholipid bilayer

A & B Intrinsic protein
C Carrier protein
D Extrinsic protein

Main Structural Features of Biomembrane

i. There is lipidous ocean enclosing proteins like the ice-bergs in ocean, so it is commonly called *lipoprotein membrane*.

ii. Lipids in membrane form lipid bilayer with the thickness 70 to 100Å.

iii. In lipid bilayer, for each lipid molecule hydrophilic or polar head is kept exposed outside. The hydrophobic or nonpolar tails for each lipid molecule are kept hidden within lipid bilayer.

iv. Proteins in the biomembrane are three main types:

    a. Extrinsic protein   c. Carrier protein

    b. Intrinsic protein

v. Extrinsic proteins are *loosely* attached to the lipid bilayer. So these proteins are easily dissociable and detachable.

vi. Intrinsic proteins are *tightly* bound to lipid bilayer and so these are not easily dissociable and detachable.

vii. Extrinsic proteins are mainly the glycoproteins and their main function is to take part in structural built up of membrane.

viii. The carrier proteins functions for in and out transport of different substances across the membrane.

Such biomembrane is described as "fluid-mosaic model":

The lipid bilayer in the membrane gives fluidity to the membrane because of specific arrangement. Proteins in the structure of biomembranes are arranged in mosaic fashion in lipid bilayer ocean. Hence this membrane structure model is described to be fluid-mosaic model.

Functions of Biomembranes

1. To perform the limiting boundary for cytoplasmic contents.
2. To control the flow of material and information in and out of the cell.
3. It forms selectively permeable barrier that allows in and to movement of some substances selectively.
4. It possess specific sites for particular chemical substances.
5. Carrier proteins of membrane functions for active transport of required substances.
6. Irritability, i.e. response at cellular level are shown by working of biomembranes.
7. Electron-transport system made up of flavoprotein called cytochromes is oxidases with biomembrane. Such ETS is required compulsory for cell respiration physiology.
8. The cilia are protoplasmic extensions and are structural part of ciliated epithelium performing specific functions in human body.

6

Enzymes

Q 1. Define enzyme. Classify enzymes into six classes with examples. (S. 97, 98, 02, 06, 09; W. 00, 02, 06, 07)

Definition

Enzymes can be defined as soluble, colloidal, organic catalysts, protein in chemical nature, produced by living cells, which accelerate the rate of reaction and working at specific pH and temperature to convert substrate into specific product.

- Enzymes are proteins which catalyse number of biochemical reactions.

Classification of Enzymes (Major 6 Classes of Enzymes)

1. *Oxidoreductases*: This class of enzyme is concerned with oxidation-reduction in which one compound is oxidised and other is reduced. Oxidation involves removal of H_2 atom or addition of oxygen, e.g. dehydrogenases, oxidases.

2. *Transferases*: These are the enzymes which catalyse transfer of chemical groups such as alkyl, methyl, carboxyl, sulphate, phosphate, aldehyde, ketone, e.g. transaminase, kinases.

3. *Hydrolyses*: This class of enzyme include hydrolytic enzymes that split different bonds such as C–N, C–O, C–C, etc. by addition of water, i.e. these enzymes catalyse hydrolytic reactions, e.g. esterases, lipases, peptidases, phosphatases, glycosidases.

4. *Lyases*: This is the 4th class of enzyme which catalyse removal of specific group from their substrate and introduce double bonds. The same enzymes can add groups to the double bonds. These enzymes catalyse the cleavage reactions which are nonhydrolytic, e.g. aldolases, decarboxylases, dehydratase, acotinoases.

5. *Isomerases*: There are the groups of enzymes which catalyse redistribution of chemical groups within a molecule to produce isomers, epimers, enantiomers, etc. They catalyse isomerization reactions, e.g. isomerases, epimerases, recemerases.

6. *Ligases*: This is the 6th class of enzymes which are called "synthetases". They catalyse the bond formation reactions, i.e. linking together of two compounds, e.g. synthetases, carboxylases.

Q 2. Mention general properties or characteristics of enzymes.

1. All enzymes are protein in chemical nature.
2. Enzymes accelerate (increase) the rate of reaction.
3. Enzymes are always specific for their substrate.
4. They posses an active site or active site at which interaction with substrate takes place.
5. In enzyme action mechanism there is a formation of enzyme-substrate complex as an important intermediate in the reaction.
6. Some enzymes are regulatory in function.
7. Enzymes are thermolabile, i.e. heat sensitive as they can be denatured or inactivate by heat.
8. Enzymes are proteins with high molecular weight ranging between 10,000 to more than millions.
9. Enzymes can be precipitated by ethanol or by high concentration of inorganic salts like NH_4SO_4.
10. Enzymes are proteins in chemical nature thus they are amphoteric, i.e. posses positive as well as negative charge due to acidic and basic functional groups.
11. Enzymes are unstable and their activity can be lowered or enzymes can be destroyed by variety of physical and chemical conditions, e.g. high temperature, wide changes in pH.

Q 3. Write in short about nomenclature of enzymes. (S. 97, 98, 02; W. 00, 02)

- Earlier for the long time enzymes were being named by adding suffix—'in', e.g. pepsin, trypsin, renin, chymotrypsin.
- Later on because of addition new enzymes nomenclature by above method becomes difficult, so enzymes can be named by new fashion, by adding suffix—'ase'.
  - i. Suffix—'ase' is added to the substrate upon which enzyme is acting, e.g. fumarase, urease, lipase, sucrase.

ii. Other way of naming enzyme by adding suffix—'ase' to the kind of reaction which is mediated by that enzyme, e.g. oxidase, reductase, transferase, ligase.

- As the number of enzymes were discovered, so there was need of systematic and informative nomenclature and classification of enzymes.

  Thus in 1961, the commission on enzymes, International Union of Biochemistry (IUB), proposed a new system of classification of enzymes.
  - The IUB formed Enzymes Commission (EC)
  - Thus the names are called EC names
  - EC names comprises of 4 digits
  - Where, first digit indicate main class
  - Second digit indicate subclass of respective main class
  - Third digit indicate main class for sub-sub-class
  - Fourth digit indicate enzyme actual.

  Example: EC 1.1.1.27 for enzyme lactate dehydrogenase (LDH).
- *Draw back*: This system is not practically usable.

Q 4. Describe in brief chemistry of enzymes.

- Some enzymes are purely protein in nature while there are certain enzymes which posses one or more nonprotein component for proper functioning of these enzymes.
- The protein part of an enzyme is called "apoenzyme" while the nonprotein part of an enzyme is called "co-factor"/"co-enzyme".
- When co-factor is firmly attached to the protein, it is called "prosthetic group".
- The active enzyme composed of apoenzyme and a co-factor is called the 'holoenzyme."

Apoenzyme   Co-factor   Holoenzyme
(protein) + (co-enzyme) ───────────────────▶ (active enzyme)

- When co-factor is not firmly (loosely) attached to the protein then it is called co-enzyme.
- There are many enzymes which requires Mg, Ca, Cu, Mn, Zn, etc. as metallic co-factor or prosthetic group.
- Some enzymes are called metalloenzymes which requires compulsory presence of metallic ion for their activity.

Q 5. Discuss different factors affecting/influencing enzyme catalysed reactions. (S. 96, 98, 99, 00, 01, 02, 04, 05, 06, 07, 09; W. 96, 97, 98, 02, 03, 04, 05, 06, 07)

   i. Effect of nature and concentration of susbstrate

   ii. Effect of nature and concentration of enzymes

  iii. Effect of time

  iv. Effect of temperature

   v. Effect of pH

  vi. Effect of UV rays

 vii. Effect of inhibitors

viii. Effect of activators

i. Effect of Nature and Concentration of Susbstrate

- If the concentration of substrate is increased by keeping concentration of enzyme constant, then rate of reaction is increased.
- Initially rate of reaction is directly proportional to substrate concentration, this is because active site of enzyme occupies substrate.
- Further increase in substrate concentration can increase the catalysis rate but when all enzyme molecules are completely occupied by substrate molecule, further increase in substrate concentration *cannot increase the rate of reaction.*
- At this state, enzymes are completely saturated with substrate.
- V_{max}: The velocity at the stage where rate of reaction is maximum is called maximum velocity. The rate of enzyme catalysed reaction is:

$$V = \frac{V_{max}\,(S)}{K_m + (S)}$$

Where, K_m = Michaelis—menten constant

     V_{max} = Maximum velocity

     (S) = Substrate concentration.

Michaelis—Menten Constant

"It is defined as the substrate concentration to which the velocity of an enzyme catalysed reaction is exactly half of V_{max}."

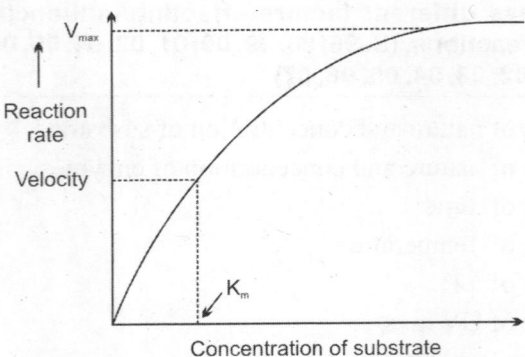

ii. **Effect of Nature and Concentration of Enzymes**

The enzyme activity is directly proportional to concentration of enzyme in the system, i.e. increase in concentration of enzyme increases the rate of reaction. It is assumed that, for increase in velocity to achieve V_{max} in the medium, substrate is present in highest concentration. Also to achieve V_{max}, the specific substrate, optimum pH and optimum temperature are to be provided.

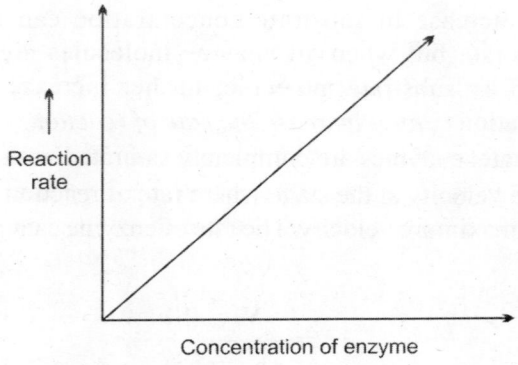

iii. **Effect of Time**

Here, a typical bell-shaped graph is obtained when reaction velocity is plotted against the time.

Initially there is rapid increase in velocity till V_{max} is achieved. After that, graph slopes down sharply as substrate concentration decreases as a resultant of enzyme catalysis, as and when time proceeds further.

The bell-shaped graph is obtained upon assumption that:
a. Both enzymes and substrates are at constant and highest concentration.
b. Optimum pH and temperature are required.

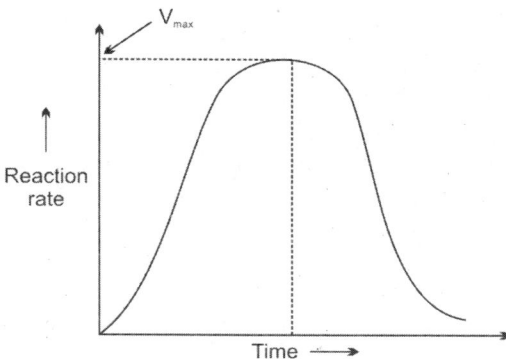

iv. **Effect of Temperature**

- The rate of enzyme catalysed reaction initially increases as the temperature increases. But this increase is obtained till optimum temperature (about 35 to 38°C).
- The temperature at which an enzyme shows maximum activity is called optimum temperature.
- Further increase in temperature decreases the velocity of enzyme catalysis and so bell-shaped graph is obtained.
- Decrease in velocity after achieving V_{max} at optimum temperature is because of thermal denaturation of enzymes. This is because proteins are destroyed or denatured at high temperature.
- The increase in temperature above the optimum temperature may result into inactivation of enzymes, this is known as thermal denaturation.

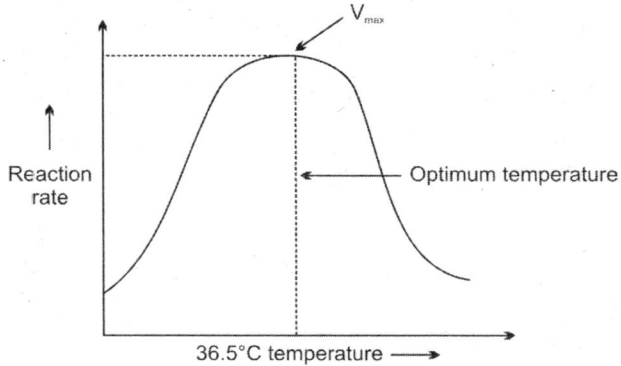

v. Effect of pH

When a graph is plotted of velocity of enzyme catalysis against pH, a typical bell-shaped graph is obtained. pH refers to acidic or basic or neutral ranges. The most of enzymes works with acidic or basic or neutral ranges. The most of the enzymes works with maximum rate at neutral pH (pH.7).

Initially increase in pH from acidic to neutral side, the velocity also increases. But upon reaching optimum pH (neutral) further increase in pH velocity of enzyme catalysis decreases significantly.

The characteristic pH at which enzyme activity is maximum is called as optimum pH.

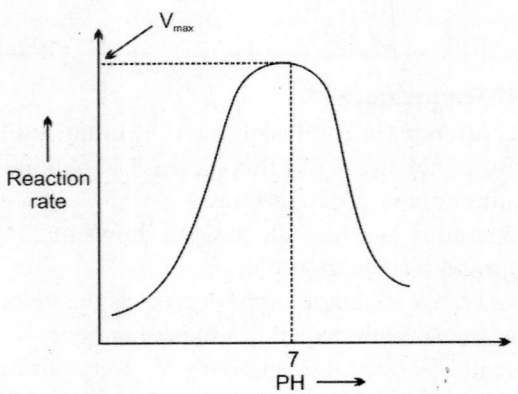

For each enzyme, there is range of optimum pH, within which enzyme work with maximum velocity. This range is generally from pH 6.4 to pH 7.5. Exceptionally there are some enzyme for which optimum pH is highly acidic or slightly acidic or alkaline are given below:

Enzyme	Optimum pH
1. Pepsin	2.0
2. Acid phosphatase	5.5
3. Papain	5 to 6
4. Amylase	6 to 7
5. Lipase	7.0
6. Trypsin	6 to 8.5
7. Alkaline phosphatase	9.2

vi. Effect of UV Rays

The UV rays affects adversely the velocity of enzyme catalysis, that is because enzymes are denatured by UV rays.

The damaging effect of UV rays is seen at highest degree at the wavelength 2650Å. It is observed that the degree of purity of enzyme decides the degree of damage of enzyme. When enzyme is with more impurities, the damaging effects of UV rays are least because impurities in enzyme absorbs UV rays with damaging effect thus protecting enzyme protein.

vii. Effect of Inhibitors

Inhibitors are the agents which prevents the action of enzyme and thus decrease the rate of reaction. Such inhibition may be by:
  i. Feedback inhibition
  ii. Competitive inhibition.

viii. Effect of Activators

Activators are the agents which increases the activity of enzyme and velocity of enzyme catalysis. The presence of enzyme activators in certain concentration increases the enzyme activity, e.g.
  i. Many enzymes require monovalent cations like K^+, Na^+ for maximum catalytic activity.
  ii. Cysteine HCl increases the proteolytic activity of papain.

Q 6. Write a note on enzyme action/mechanism of enzyme action/concept of enzyme action. (S. 96, 97, 98, 99, 01, 03, 05, 06, 07; W. 02, 06)

- Enzymes are biological catalyst which act upon substrate to convert it into the end product.
- Enzymes mainly works to accelerate the rate of reaction.
- In 1913, Michaelis and Menten established the theory of formation of an enzyme-substrate complex and its subsequent dissociation into products.
- In actual mechanism of catalysis, enzymes initially forms a complex with substrate molecule called as enzyme-substrate complex.

Enzyme (E) + Substrate (S) $\longrightarrow$ Enzyme-substrate complex
(ES complex)

ES $\longrightarrow$ E + Product (P)

- The binding sites on the enzyme molecules having competitive structures to the substrate molecule so that they can 'fit' into particular site on an enzyme molecule.
- The binding of a substrate with an enzyme at the active site, is explained by two theories.
  - i. Lock and key hypothesis/model
  - ii. Induced fit hypothesis.

i. Lock and Key Hypothesis (Emil Fischer)

- It is the first ever idea proposed by scientist "Emil Fischer" to explain enzyme action mechanism. It is like a lock and key.
- In this case, the shape of active site of enzyme and that of substrate is complementary to each other.
- The substrate molecule fits into the active site of an enzyme just as a key fits into a lock. Hence this type of mechanism is termed as lock and key model/hypothesis.
- In this model, the shape of the active site is rigid and complementary to the shape of the substrate complex.
- Mechanism:

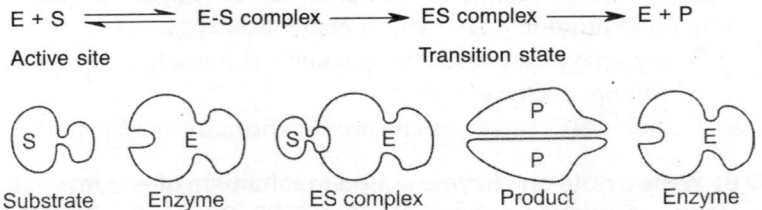

Limitations/Drawbacks of Lock and Key Hypothesis

  i. Rigid structure of enzyme as stated in this hypothesis is not exactly proved. Infact enzymes being protein in nature possess structural flexibility, because of changes in coiling and recoiling of polypeptide chain in enzyme protein.
  ii. For one enzyme acting upon one class of substrate, lock and key hypothesis fails, e.g. enzyme lipase acting upon lipids and fats in general, from different sources and with different chemical natures.

ii. Induced Fit Model/Hypothesis (S. 08)

- It is the hypothesis proposed by scientist Koshland, where limitations of lock and key hypothesis are removed.

- Induced fit hypothesis states that in an unoccupied enzyme molecule functional group of active site are not in their optimum position to promote catalysis, i.e. shape of active site is not complementary to the substrate.
- In this hypothesis, the active site of an enzyme is considerably flexible so as to accommodate a wide variety of susbtrate molecule.
- Thus when substrate molecule binds to the enzyme, the shape of active site is made complementary to the substrate to certain extent.
- The hypothesis is called induced fit because the substrate molecule that induce enzyme to undergo favourable confirmation (changes).

1.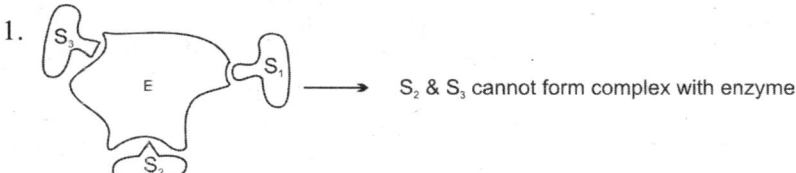

S_2 & S_3 cannot form complex with enzyme

2.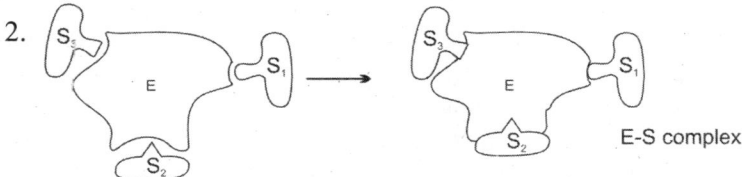

E-S complex

Active site of enzyme is made complementary as that of shape of the substrate.

In actual mechanism following steps are important:

a. Favourable proximity and orientation between both substrate and enzyme.

b. Covalent catalysis by covalent bond formation between substrate and enzyme at active site.

c. Several group of enzyme (acid-base reaction) forms main basis of enzyme action mechanism.

Q 7. What is enzyme inhibition? Discuss the different types of enzyme inhibition/Write a note on enzyme inhibition. (S. 01; W. 96, 97, 98, 01, 05, 07)

Enzyme Inhibition

The functional groups of enzymes from their active sites and surfaces react with a variety of chemical agents and their catalytic activity is reduced. These agents are called as inhibitors and the process is called as enzyme inhibition.

Types of Enzyme Inhibition

a. *Competitive inhibition or reversible inhibition*

   i. In this type of inhibition, the inhibitors have structural similarity with the substrate.
   ii. Due to this the inhibitors binds at the active site of enzyme.
   iii. In this case, the inhibitors and substrate both are competing for the active of an enzyme. Hence it is called as competitive inhibition.
   iv. If the concentration of substrate increased then the inhibition can be reversed, hence called reversible inhibition.
   v. Inhibitors bind with the enzyme to form an enzyme inhibitors complex which does not give a product.

$$E + S \rightleftharpoons ES \longrightarrow E + P$$

$$E + I \rightleftharpoons EI \longrightarrow \text{No product}$$

   vi. Example: Malonic acid is a competitive inhibitors of enzyme succinic acid dehydrogenase because there is a structural similarity between malonic and succinic acid.
   vii. The K_m value of enzyme increases in the presence of competition inhibition and V_{max} remains constant.

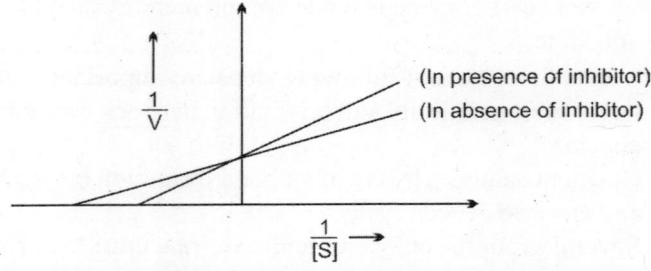

   viii. Other examples of competitive inhibitors:
   - Allopurinol is a competitive inhibitors of xanthine oxidase.
   - Ephedrine is a competitive inhibitors of mono-amino oxidase enzyme.

b. *Noncompetitive inhibition/irreversible inhibition*

   i. In this type of inhibition, inhibitors binds with an enzyme at the surface of functional group and reduce the activity of enzyme. Thus increase in substrate concentration does not reverse inhibition.

ii. In this case the inhibitor can also be bound to the enzyme substrate complex.

$$E + S \rightleftharpoons ES \longrightarrow E + P$$

$$E + I \rightleftharpoons EI \longrightarrow \text{No product}$$

$$ES + I \rightleftharpoons ESI \longrightarrow \text{No product}$$

$$EI + S \rightleftharpoons EIS \longrightarrow \text{No product}$$

iii. The K_m value of an enzyme remains constant but V_{max} decreases.

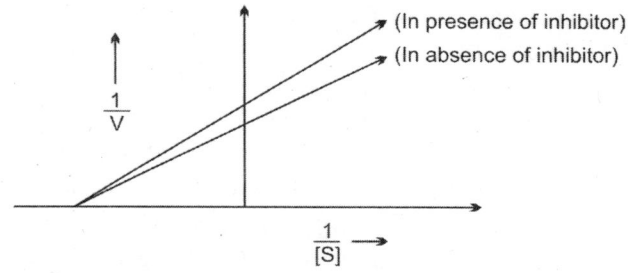

iv. Examples of noncompetitive inhibitor: Metal ions and EDTA shows noncompetitive inhibition.

Q 8. Differences (S. 06)

Competitive inhibition	Noncompetitive inhibition
i. The inhibitors have a structural similarity with the substrate.	i. No structural relationship between inhibitors and substrate.
ii. The inhibitors binds at the active site of an enzyme.	ii. The inhibitors binds with an enzyme at surface of functional group.
iii. The increase in substrate concentration decreases inhibition.	iii. The increase in susbtrate concentration does not decrease inhibition.
iv. K_m value of enzyme increases in presence of competitive inhibition.	iv. The K_m value of an enzyme remain constant.

Contd.

Competitive inhibition	Non-competitive inhibition
v. V_{max} value remain constant.	v. V_{max} value decreases.
vi. This is called reversible inhibition.	vi. This is called irreversible inhibition.
vii. Examples: Ephedrine is a competitive inhibitor of MAO enzymes.	vii. Examples: Metal ions and EDTA shows non-competitive inhibition.

Q 9. Define the terms with examples.

1. *Cofactor*: Some enzymes requires a nonprotein group for catalytic activity which is called as cofactor, e.g. the metal ions like Mg^{++}, Mn^{++}, Ca^{++} are called as cofactors.

2. *Coenzymes*: Coenzymes are low-molecular weight organic substances essentially derived from vitamin B complex group and are required for catalytic reactions, e.g. pyridoxal phosphate is derived from vitamin B_6, which is a co-enzyme of transaminase.

3. *Endoenzymes/intracellular enzymes*: The enzymes which acts only inside the cell and involve in synthesis of cell components, food material of the cell, are known as *endoenzymes*, e.g. synthetase, isomerases.

4. *Exoenzymes/extracellular enzymes*: The enzymes which are secured outside the cell having a digestive function are called exoenzymes, e.g. pepsin, lipase, amylase, trypsin.

5. *Constitutive enzymes*: The enzymes which are produced in the absence of substrate are called as constitutive enzymes, e.g. enzymes of glycolytic series such as kinase, mutase.

6. *Induced enzymes*: The enzymes which are present in small amount but their concentration get immediately increased in the presence of substrate on which they act. Such enzymes are called as induced enzymes, e.g. ethanol and barbiturates are powerful in inducing hepatic microsomal enzymes.

7. *Holoenzyme*: The active enzyme composed of apoenzyme and a cofactor is called holoenzyme.

$$\text{Apoenzyme + Cofactor} \longrightarrow \text{Holoenzyme}$$

8. *Apoenzyme*: The protein part of an enzyme is called apoenzyme.

9. *Isoenzymes*: The multiple forms of the same enzyme are called isoenzymes, e.g. lactate dehydrogenase (LDH).

10. *Proenzymes/zymogens*: The enzymes which are present in its inactive forms are called as proenzymes, e.g. pepsinogen, trypsinogen.

11. *Activators* (*enzymes activators*): Some enzymes requires presence of small amounts of specific inorganic ions for their activity. Such ions are called as activators.

These ions may help in joining with groups on the susbtrate molecule and bringing them together with enzymes or by actual participation in transfer reaction.

   i. Mg^{++} ions required for phosphorylation reaction

   ii. Ca^{++} ions required for coagulation

   iii. Zn^{++} ions required for carbonic anhydrase action

   iv. Fe^{++} and Cu^{++} ions required for some oxidative reaction.

12. *Active site*: It is a cleft or depression upon enzyme molecule at which substrate molecule attaches to enzyme. Enzyme molecule may carry one or many active sites.

13. *Enzymes inhibitors*: The functional groups of enzymes from their active sites and surfaces reaction with a variety of chemical reagents and their catalytic activity is reduced. These agents are called enzymes inhibitors, e.g. ephedrine is an inhibitor of MAO enzymes.

14. *Allosteric enzymes*: The enzymes whose catalytic activity is regulated by itself are called allosteric enzymes. These are also called as regulatory enzymes, e.g. phosphofructokinase is an allosteric enzymes which convert fructose-6-phosphate to fructose-1,6-diphosphate.

Q 10. Write a short note on zymogen's/proenzymes. (S. 96, 98, 01, 02; W. 08)

Definition

Some enzymes which are present in its inactive form are called as zymogens or proenzymes.

• Proenzyme is synthesized in the inactive state.

• Subsequently proenzyme is activated and converted to the active enzyme form in the presence of some molecules or factors called as activators.

- Typically protein digesting enzymes and blood coagulation factors are synthesized in their zymogen form.

- Examples:

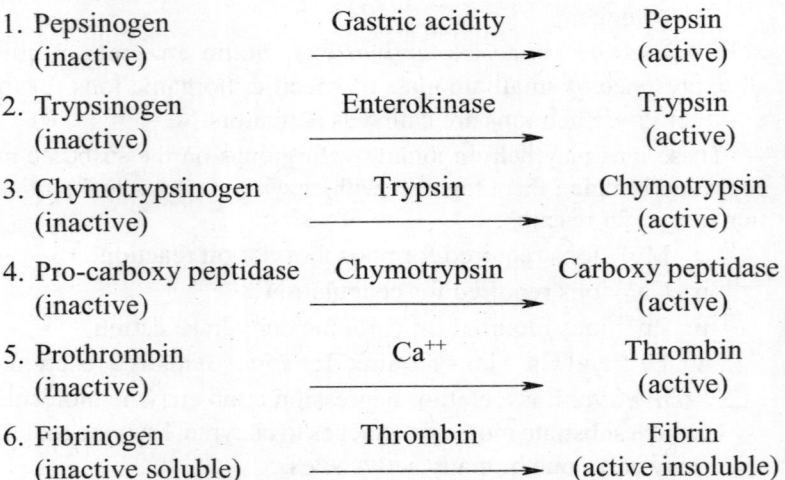

1. Pepsinogen (inactive) → [Gastric acidity] → Pepsin (active)

2. Trypsinogen (inactive) → [Enterokinase] → Trypsin (active)

3. Chymotrypsinogen (inactive) → [Trypsin] → Chymotrypsin (active)

4. Pro-carboxy peptidase (inactive) → [Chymotrypsin] → Carboxy peptidase (active)

5. Prothrombin (inactive) → [Ca^{++}] → Thrombin (active)

6. Fibrinogen (inactive soluble) → [Thrombin] → Fibrin (active insoluble)

Example of Proenzyme Activation

- Pepsinogen is a zymogen form of protein digesting enzyme pepsin.
- This enzyme is present in gastric juice in the stomach.
- Free HCl secreted by stomach mucosa works as activator to convert inactive pepsinogen to active pepsin.
- Action of HCl results in cutting and removal of a fragment of 45 amino acids present at N-terminal of inactive pepsinogen. This changes conformation of enzyme protein molecule to convert inactive pepsinogen to active pepsin.

Significance of Zymogens

Till particular proenzyme is activated, particular enzyme cannot operate in the body, e.g. damage of gastric and intestinal mucosa can be prevented by protein digesting enzymes secreted in respective zymogen form. In another example by secreting some blood clotting factors in zymogen form clotting of circulating blood in the body is prevented. Blood clot in circulating blood (thrombus) can block blood vessels thus to prevent blood supply and further damage, some blood clotting factors are produced in zymogen forms.

Q 11. Write a note no isoenzymes/isozymes. (S. 96, 98, 01, 02; W. 07)

Isoenzymes

The enzymes which have multiple molecular forms in the same organism and catalysing same biochemical reactions are called isoenzymes/isozymes.

The multiple forms of the same enzyme are called as isoenzymes. Isoenzymes, though catalyse same reaction, they differ in degree of activity show, i.e. V_{max} for different isoenzymes is different. Relative amounts of different forms of isoenzymes differ in different organs and tissues.

Examples of Isoenzymes

1. LDH, i.e. lactate dehydrogenase in five different forms.
2. Alkaline phosphatase in two different forms.
3. Isocitrate dehydrogenase in three different forms.
4. Creatinine phosphokinase in three different forms.

   Creatinine phosphokinase (CPK) is isoenzyme with three different forms as:
   a. CPK-1 BB
   b. CPK-2 BM
   c. CPK-3 MM.

   Where in these three forms are polypeptide chain in the enzyme protein is denoted by 'B' and other polypeptide chain is denoted by 'M'.

Q 12. Write in brief about lactate dehydrogenase (LDH).

* LDH is the most important enzyme existing in almost all tissues and body fluids in the human body.
* This enzyme catalyse dehydrogenation reaction, i.e. removal of hydrogen to convert lactic acid into pyruvic acid.

$$\text{Lactate} + NAD^+ \xrightarrow{\text{Lactate dehydrogenase}} \text{Pyruvate} + NADH + H^+$$

* As a part of tissue respiration physiology in all the cell, certain amount of LDH is present.
* Following are five different isoenzyme forms of LDH with their respective subunits as:

  LDH_1—H_4 Where two polypeptides are indicated by
  LDH_2—$H_3 M$ H and M.

LDH_3—$H_2 M_2$

LDH_4—HM_3

LDH_5—M_4

- LDH is most important glycolytic enzyme present in nearly all the cells but higher concentration is seen in:
  - Liver (LDH_5—60%)
  - Skeletal muscles (LDH_5—55%)
  - Heart (myocardium) (LDH_1—55%) (LDH_2—36%)
  - Kidney (LDH_5—45%)
  - Brain (LDH_5—40%), (LDH_1 and LDH_2 both about 20%).
- The pattern of distribution of particular type of LDH isoenzyme possess clinical or diagnostic value.

  The disturbance and the increase in serum LDH level is seen in muscular dystrophy, kidney disease, haemolytic anaemia, megaloblastic anaemia and in different types of cancer.
- Normal value of serum LDH is 60 to 200 IU/litre.

Q 13. What is marker enzyme? Write a note on marker enzyme. (S. 99, 00, 01; W. 00)

Marker Enzyme

Marker enzymes are that enzymes which gives signals and are helpful in transportation.

- These are recognised by the specific DNA sequence.
- The soluble enzymes of citric acid cycle and β-oxidation of fatty acid found in matrix, are necessary for transporting metabolites and nucleotides across the inner membrane.
- Succinate dehydrogenase is found on the inner surface of the inner mitochondrial membrane.
- The cell organelles and relative marker enzymes are as follows:

Cell organelles	Marker enzymes
i. Nucleus	DNA polymerase
ii. Mitochondria	Glutamic dehydrogenase
iii. Endoplasmic reticulum	Glucose-6-phosphate
iv. Golgi apparatus	Galactosyl transferase.

Functions of Marker Enzymes

  i. They gives signals and are helpful in transportation.

ii. They helps to transport metabolites and nucleotides across the inner membrane.

iii. Marker enzymes have diagnostic value, e.g. during infection, the leakage of marker enzyme increases. Hence such increase of certain enzymes from plasma is used for diagnosis of diseases.

Q 14. What is transaminase? Give the diagnostic applications of it. (W. 97)

Definition

The enzymes which are involved in transamination reaction in living organism are called transaminases.

There are two types of transaminase fund in human tissues:

i. GOT (Glutamate oxaloacetic transaminase)

ii. GPT (Glutamate pyruvic transaminase).

• The transaminase are widely distributed in nature.

• GOT in present in greatest amount in heart muscles, skeletal muscles, brain, liver, and kidney.

• Traces of these enzymes normally escapes into the blood stream.

• The normal level of SGOT and SGPT are:

SGOT—2 to 30 IU/litre

SGPT—2 to 15 IU/litre.

Diagnostic Applications of Transaminase

i. In myocardial infarction, SGOT level is increased.

ii. Damage of small portion of heart muscle by occlusion of branch of coronary arteries may increase SGOT level.

iii. In rural hepatitis SGPT is always higher than SGOT.

iv. In cirrhosis and demolytic jaundice SGOT is higher than SGPT.

v. Increased SGOT level in skeletal muscles indicates damage or injury to skeletal muscle and also muscular dystrophy.

Q 15. Write in brief about medicinal significance of enzymes.

Many drugs exert their actions by inhibiting certain enzyme systems. Hence enzyme inhibition has a great significance in the treatment of diseases, these are:

i. Sulfanilamide selectively kills pathogenic organisms by inhibiting 'folic acid synthetase' enzyme.

ii. Ephedrine is a competitive inhibitor of mono-amino oxidase enzyme and prolongs the action of mono-amines and exerts an antidepressant activity.

iii. Allopurinol is a competitive inhibitor of xanthine oxidase enzyme. Hence allopurinol is used in the treatment of gout.

Q 16. Give therapeutic and pharmaceutical importance of enzymes. (S. 98, 99, 00, 02, 03, 05, 08, 09; W. 96, 99, 00, 02)

1. Therapeutic Importance of Enzymes

Enzymes are frequently used therapeutically, these are:

a. The enzyme L-asparaginase is used in treatment of cancer.

b. Galactosidase can be used for the treatment of lactose intolerance in children.

c. Fibrinolysin and deoxyribonuclease may help to remove fibrinous material from infected wounds.

d. Trypsin, streptokinase enzymes are used in the treatment of thrombosis.

e. Pepsin, lipase, amylase, peptidases are used in the treatment of chronic pancreatitis and gastrointestinal disorders.

2. Therapeutic Importance of Enzymes (In Manufacturing of Bulk Drugs)

Some enzymes are used in bulk drug manufacturing.

i. Penicillin acylase is used for the production of 6-amino-penicillanic acid from penicillin-G.

ii. Papain is used as digestant for the production of protein hydrolysates.

iii. Hyaluronidase is used in orthopaedic practice.

iv. Urokinase is used in cardiac diseases.

v. Amino acylase for production of L-amino acids.

vi. Glucose isomerase is used for production of high fructose syrup.

vii. Amylase is used for production of dextrin.

Q 17. Give the diagnostic uses/significance of enzymes. (S. 01; W. 07)

The enzymatic pattern is different for different tissues in higher animals. Hence enzymes have a great value in the diagnosis of diseases.

Examples

  i. 'Aspartate aminotransferase' and 'lactate dehydrogenase' are seen in cardiac and hepatic tissues and helps in the diagnosis of 'myocardial infarction' and 'hepatitis'.

 ii. 'Creatine kinase' is seen in skeletal or cardiac muscles and helps in diagnosis of skeletal or cardiac disorders.

iii. In some pathological condition the enzyme amylase is found to be released in blood circulation, e.g. damage to gland cells and damage to secretary pathway.

 iv. The increase in serum aldolase level shows some important disease like, myocardial infarction, viral hepatitis, liver cancer.

  v. Human plasma contains a wide range of enzymes. During infection, the leakage of marker enzyme increases. Hence such increase of certain enzyme from plasma is used for the diagnosis of diseases.

7

Vitamins and Coenzymes

Q 1. Define vitamins. Give the classification of vitamins. (S. 96, 97, 01, 02, 03, 04, 05, 06, 09; W. 98, 01, 02)

Vitamins

Vitamins are the organic compounds which are found in natural food stuffs and are essential for normal growth and metabolic functions of the body.

Classification of Vitamins

- *Fat soluble vitamins*: Vitamin A, vitamin D, vitamin E, vitamin K.
- *Water soluble vitamins*:
  - i. Vitamin B complex group
    - Thiamine (B_1)
    - Riboflavin (B_2)
    - Niacin (B_3)
    - Pyridoxine (B_6)
    - Pantothenic acid
    - Biotin
    - Folic acid
    - Lipolic acid (PABA)
    - Cyanocobalamin.
  - ii. Ascorbic acid (vitamin C).

Q 2. Explain the terms.

a. *Night blindness*: It is an ability to have vision in dim light and during dark, due to impairment in dark adaptation of eyes.

It is caused due to deficiency of vitamin A.

In children, additional defects like recurrent infection and diarrhoea may observe.

b. *Pellagra* (*S. 98, 01, 06, 08; W. 07*): It is caused due to deficiency of niacin (vitamin B_3)
   - *Symptoms*:
     i. Dermatitis
     ii. A sore
     iii. Dark coloured tongue
     iv. An inability to digest and assimilate food
     v. Skin rash, itching.

c. *Scurvy* (*W. 07*): It is a deficiency disorder caused due to vitamin C.
   - *Symptoms*:
     i. Defective formation of collagen fibres of connective tissues
     ii. Formation of bone is also abnormal
     iii. Bleeding occurs
     iv. Pin-point haemorrhages in the skin
     v. Bleeding from gums and teeth
     vi. Slow wound healing
     vii. Slow healing of fractured bones.

d. *Egg white injury* (*W. 07*): It is a deficiency disorder caused due to vitamin 'biotin'. Biotin has a strong affinity with avidin (egg white protein). Excess consumption of raw eggs result in deficiency of biotin called as egg white injury.

   This biotin-avidin complex is not absorbed during digestion and hence produces deficiency of biotin.
   - *Symptoms*:
     i. Nausea
     ii. Anorexia
     iii. Dermatitis
     iv. Pains in muscles
     v. Fatigue.

Q 3. Write a note on beriberi. (S. 04; W. 06, 07)

Beriberi

It is a deficiency disorder of vitamin B_1 (thiamine). There are four types of beriberi.

a. *Dry beriberi:* It is a nutritional deficiency. The main reason behind this is consumption of polished rice and refined cereals.
   - *Symptoms*:
     i. Degeneration and demyelination
     ii. Oedema of face and legs

    iii. Pericardial pains

    iv. Palpitation

    v. Numbness in legs

    vi. Tenderness in the calf muscles.

b. *Wet beriberi:* It is characterized by oedema. Reason behind oedema is cardiac failure.

* *Symptoms*:

    i. Rapid and notable oedema develops involving face, legs, trunk and serous cavities

    ii. Breathlessness

    iii. Palpitation

    iv. Rise in systolic BP

    v. The severe condition patient may die due to acute circulatory failure.

c. *Infantile beriberi:* It occurs in breastfed infants, usually between 2 to 5 months of age. Reason behind is mother consuming thiamine deficient diet and secreting milk with low thiamine content. It is very acute condition and can be fatal (toxic).

* *Symptoms*:

    i. Restlessness in infants

    ii. Infant crises a lot and passes very less urine

    iii. Oedema develops

    iv. Dyspnoea

    v. Tachycardia

    vi. Infant may die within 24 to 48 hours

    vii. Convulsions and coma.

d. *Cerebral beriberi:* This disease is resultant of acute biochemical lesions in the brain due to thiamine deficient diet. It is further leading to abnormal metabolism in the brain:

* *Reason behind cerebral beriberi*

    i. Alcoholism

    ii. Carcinoma in stomach

    iii. Pregnancy toxaemia

    iv. Prolonged vomiting

    v. Diarrhoea.

* *Symptoms*:

    i. Vomiting

    ii. Psychiatric disorders like disorientation, faulty memory

iii. Loss of pupillary reflex
iv. Loss of extraocular movements
v. Polyneuritis.

Q 4. Give biological role/functions and deficiency disorders of vitamin A. (S. 00, 01, 03, 09; W. 98, 00, 01, 02, 03)

Functions of Vitamin A

* Vitamin A is the structural part of retinal pigment called as "rhodopsin".
* It is required compulsory to obtain proper vision mainly during dark (dim light).
* Vitamin A keeps the mucous membranes healthy.
* Vitamin A maintains integrity and normal working of epithelial tissues and glands in the body.
* Vitamin A supports normal growth of skeleton (bones and cartilages).
* Vitamin A shows anti-infection action, protecting body against diseases caused by microbes.
* Sometimes vitamin A shows protective effect against some cancers of epithelial tissues, e.g. bronchial asthma.

Deficiency Defects of Vitamin A

i. Night blindness
ii. Conjunctival xerosis
iii. Bitots spot
iv. Corneal xerosis
v. Keratomalacia.

Extraocular Manifestations

i. Follicular hyperketosis
ii. Anorexia
iii. Retarded growth
iv. Weakness towards respiratory and intestinal infections
v. Abnormal changes in the skin.

Q 5. Give biological role/functions and deficiency disorders of vitamin D. (S. 03, 04; W. 96, 98, 99, 02, 08)

Functions of Vitamin D

* It promotes absorption of calcium of phosphorus by mucosa of small intestine.

- It also increase renal absorption of calcium and phosphorus.
- It promotes normal growth and development of bones.
- In adult stage it is required to maintain bones in healthy condition.
- It allows maturation of collagen and collagenous tissue.
- It stimulates and promotes overall normal growth of the body.

Deficiency Defects of Vitamin D

  i. Rickets in children
 ii. Osteomalacia
iii. Osteoporosis
 iv. Hypocalcaemia.

Q 6. Give biological role and deficiency disorders of vitamin C. (S. 98, 01, 03; W. 99, 02)

Functions of Vitamin C

- It keeps the gums and teeth healthy.
- It is necessary for normal tissue oxidation physiology.
- It is required for synthesis of collagen in all connective tissues.
- It reduces iron, allowing iron absorption by mucosa of small intestine.
- It provides protection against infections, so it is sometimes called anti-infective vitamin.
- It is required for separation and absorption of iron from complex sources of vegetarian food.
- It acts as a coenzyme for enzymes catalysed reactions.
- It helps in wound healing process.

Deficiency Disorders of Vitamin C

Scurvy.

Q 7. Give biological role and deficiency disorders of folic acid. (S. 98, 01; W. 99)

Functions of Folic Acid

- Folic acid is a coenzymes for the synthesis of purine and pyrimidines.
- Folic acid is required for synthesis of DNA and RNA.
- Folic aid is needed to promote rapid cell division to cause growth and development.
- It is required for erythropoiesis which occurs in bone marrow, i.e. process of formation of RBCs.

Deficiency Defect of Folic Acid

   i. Megaloblastic anaemia

  ii. Glossitis

Q 8. Give the functions and deficiency defects of vitamin B_{12} (cyanocobalamin).

Functions of Vitamin B_{12}

- Along with folic acid, vitamin B_{12} is required for normal development and maturation of RBCs.
- It is helpful in many biochemical reactions as coenzyme.
- It plays role in synthesis of fatty acids in myelin sheath of myelinated nerve fibres.
- Vitamin B_{12} acts as a coenzyme is methyl group transfer reactions.
- Vitamin B_{12} is required for conversion of RNA into DNA.

Deficiency Disorders of Vitamin B_{12}

Pernicious anaemia.

Q 9. Give the physiological functions and deficiency of riboflavin (vitamin B_2). (S. 98, 99)

Functions of Riboflavin

- It is most important constituent of flavoprotein.
- It is required as coenzyme for tissue oxidation and cellular respiration.
- It helps to carry out proper metabolisms of carbohydrates proteins and fats.
- It protect normal growth and development.
- It is required for proper maintenance of skin, oral mucosa and for normal condition of eye.

Deficiency Symptoms of Riboflavin

    i. Corneal vascularization

   ii. Angular stomatitis

  iii. Reddening of lips and tissues at the corner of mouth

  iv. Sensation of itching

   v. Burning of eyelids

  vi. Dermatitis.

Q 10. Name the vitamin along with their deficiency disorders. (W. 96)

Vitamins	Deficiency diseases
Vitamin A	Night blindness, xerophthalmia
Vitamin D	Rickets, osteomalacia
Vitamin K	Impaired blood clotting
Vitamin E	Anacondas
Vitamin B_1 (Thiamine)	Beriberi
Vitamin B_2 (Riboflavin)	Skin lesion
Vitamin B_3 (Niacin)	Pellagra
Vitamin B_6 (Pyridoxine)	Dermatitis
Vitamin M (Folic acid)	Megaloblastic anaemia
Vitamin B_{12} (Cyanocobalamin)	Pernicious anaemia
Vitamin C (Ascorbic acid)	Scurvy
Biotin	Egg white injury

Q 11. What are coenzymes? Give the coenzymes of respective vitamins. (S. 98, 04, 08; W. 04, 07)

Coenzymes: Coenzymes are organic compounds which are covalently bound to enzyme protein and are responsible for catalytic activity of several enzymes.

Coenzymes are generally derived from the water soluble B-complex vitamins and carry out transfer of hydrogen or any other group of substrate in an enzymatic reaction. Following are the list of coenzymes with their respective vitamins and their functions.

Vitamins	Coenzymes	Functions
Riboflavin (B_2)	FAD, FMN	Transfer of hydrogen
Niacin (B_3)	NAD^+ NADP	Transfer of hydrogen
Thiamine (B_1)	TPP	Transfer of acetaldehyde
Biotin	Biotin	Transfer in carbohxylation
Pyridoxine (B_6)	Pyridoxal phosphate	Transfer of amino group
Folic acid	THF	Transfer acyl group
Pantothenic acid	CoA	Transfer acyl group

8

Normal and Abnormal Metabolism

Q 1. Define metabolism. Give its importance. (W. 97)

Metabolism

Metabolism is a process in which number of biochemical changes occurs in a body and helps in exchange of matter and energy between cell and its environment.

Importance of Metabolism

i. Chemical energy is obtained.
ii. Dietary nutrients are used for synthesis of new molecules.
iii. New molecule unit to forms proteins, nucleic acids, etc.

Q 2. Define the terms. (S. 96, 02, 03, 04, 05, 07, 08, 09; W. 96, 99, 05, 08)

i. *Catabolism*: It is the degradative phase of metabolism which provides metabolic fuel and building blocks for the cell.

ii. *Anabolism*: It is the process by which the absorbed food helps in the formation of new cells, new molecules and structural and functional units of cell and essential metabolites, is known as anabolism.

iii. *Abnormal metabolism*: The metabolic process where there are deficiencies of enzymes and produce inborn errors of metabolism. This is called abnormal metabolism.

 • *Reasons for abnormal metabolism*
   i. Genetic defect
   ii. Dietary deficiencies
   iii. Diseased condition.

Q 3. What is ATP? Give its role in biological systems.

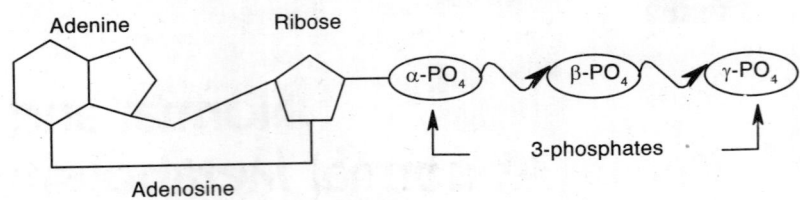

- ATP is adenosine triphosphate.
- It is a complex compound consisting of purine base-adenine, a 50 carbon sugar—the ribose, and three molecules of phosphate.
- ATP is a high energy releasing compound.

Importance of ATP

1. ATP provides energy for the synthesis of carbohydrases.
2. ATP is the main sources of energy for various metabolic activities.

Q 4. Define the terms. (S. 98, 05, 06, 07, 08, 09; W. 03, 04, 05)

  i. *Glycogenesis*: It is the process of conversion of glucose into glycogen in the liver.
 ii. *Glycogenolysis*: It is the process of breakdown of glycogen into glucose in the liver.
iii. *Gluconeogenesis/neoglucogenesis*: It is the process of synthesis of glucose from noncarbohydrates sources such as amino acids, lactic acid and glycerol, etc.
 iv. *Glycolysis*: It is the pathway in which glucose is broken down through a series of chemical reactions leading to formation of pyruvic acid

Q 5. Give the schematic representation of glycolysis/EMP pathway. (S. 97, 01, 02, 06; W. 96, 99, 00, 01, 02, 03, 04, 05, 07, 08)

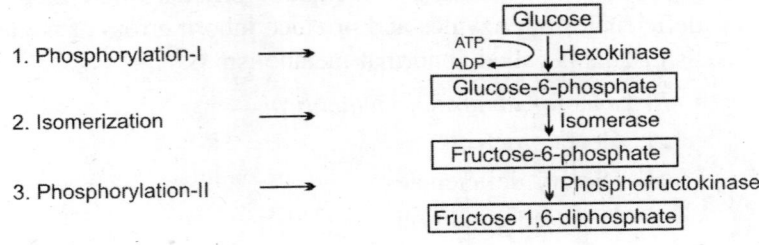

1. Phosphorylation-I ⟶
2. Isomerization ⟶
3. Phosphorylation-II ⟶

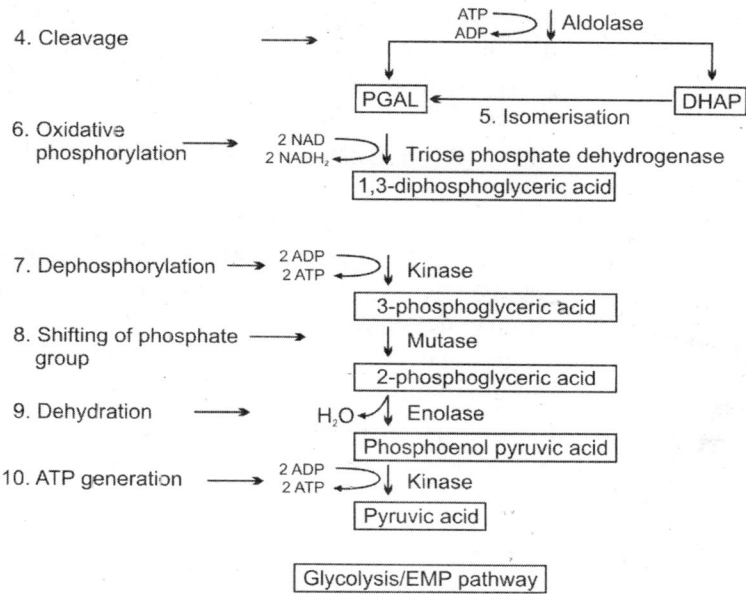

Glucolysis

Explanation

Glycolysis is the pathway in which glucose is broken down through a series of chemical reactions leading to formation of pyruvic acid.

Reactions involved in glycolysis are as follows:

1. *Phosphorylation-I*: In this reaction glucose is converted into glucose-6-phosphate in the presence of enzyme hexokinase. At this stage one ATP is converted into ADP.

2. *Isomerization*: In this reaction glucose-6-phosphate is converted into fructose-6-phosphate in the presence of isomerase enzyme.

3. *Phosphorylation-II*: Fructose-6-phosphate undergo phosphorylation with ATP and form fructose-1,6-diphosphate in the presence of enzyme phosphofructokinase.

4. *Cleavage*: In this reaction fructose-1,6-diphosphate splits into phosphoglyceraldehyde (PGAL) and dihydroxy acetone phosphate (DHAP) in the presence of enzyme aldolase.

5. *Isomerization*: DHAP is further undergo isomerization to form PGAL.

6. *Oxidative phoshorylation*: PGAL is converted into 1,3-diphosphoglyceric acid in the presence of enzyme triose phosphate dehydrogenase. In this stage 2 NAD is converted into 2 $NADH_2$.

7. *Dephosphorylation*:In this reaction, 1,3-diphosphoglyceric acid is converted into 3-phosphoglyceric acid by removal of one phosphate group.
   In this stage 2 ADP are converted into 2 ATP.

8. *Shifting of phosphate group*: In this reaction phosphate group from 3-phosphoglyceric acid is shifted to carbon number 2 in the presence of enzyme mutase.

9. *Dehydration*: 2-phosphoglyceric acid after dehydration produce phosphoenol pyruvic acid in the presence of enzyme enolase.

10. *Formation of pyruvic acid*: Phosphoenol pyruvic acid is converted into pyruvic acid in the presence of enzyme kinase. At this stage 2 ATP molecules are synthesized.

Energetics of Glycolysis

Reaction	ATP formed
1. Oxidative phosphorylation	06
2. Dephosphorylation	02
3. Phosphoenol pyruvic acid to pyruvic acid	02
Total	10 ATP
ATP consumed in:	
1. Phosphorylation-I	01
2. Phosphorylation-II	01
Total	02 ATP

Thus, in glycolysis (10 – 2 = 08) ATPs are synthesized.

Q 6. Write a note on Krebs cycle/TCA cycle/citric acid cycle. (S. 96, 98, 99, 00, 02, 04, 05, 06, 07, 08; W. 97, 98, 99, 06, 08)

Definition

The cycle of reactions involved in the oxidation of acetyl CoA into CO_2 and H_2O are collectively called as Krebs cycle, as it is discovered by Sir Han's Krebs.

In this cycle, different tricarboxylic acids are formed hence called as tricarboxylic acid cycle (TCA cycle).

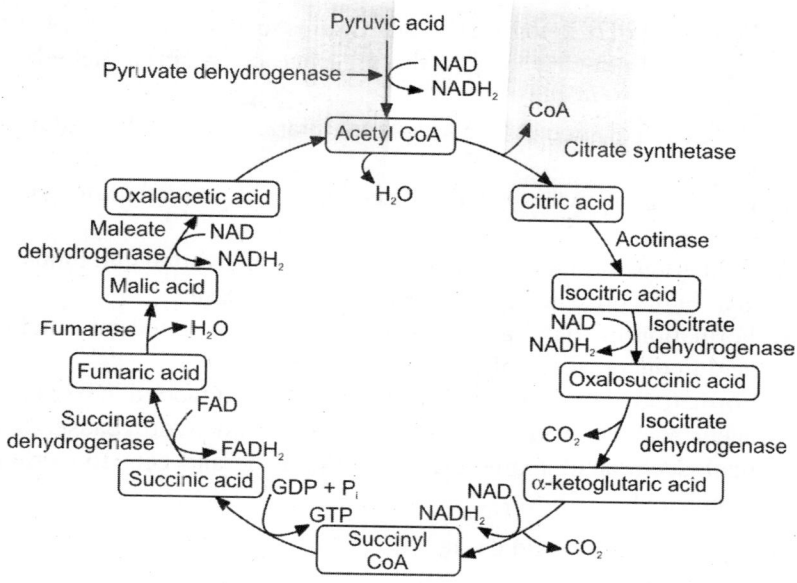

Reactions

1. Formation of acetyl CoA
2. Formation of isocitric acid
3. Formation of oxalosuccinic acid
4. Formation of α-ketoglutaric acid
5. Formation of succinyl CoA
6. Formation of succinic acid
7. Formation of fumaric acid
8. Formation of malic acid
9. Formation of oxaloacetic acid.

Krebs Cycle

1. Formation of acetyl CoA: Pyruvic acid is decarboxylated to acetyl CoA for its entry into citric acid cycle. In this stage NAD is converted into $NADH_2$.

2. Formation of isocitric acid: Acetyl CoA is converted into citric acid which further converted into isocitric acid in the presence of enzyme acotinase.

3. Formation of oxalosuccinic acid: Isocitric acid gets converted into oxalosuccinic acid in the presence of enzyme isocitrate dehydrogenase.

4. Formation of α-ketoglutaric acid: Oxalosuccinic acid is converted into α-ketoglutaric acid in the presence of isocitrate dehydrogenase.
5. Formation of succinyl CoA: α-ketoglutaric acid is converted into succinyl CoA.
6. Formation of succinic acid: Succinyl CoA is converted into succinic acid.
7. Formation of fumaric acid: Succinic acid is converted into fumaric acid in the presence of succinate dehydrogenase.
8. Formation of malic acid: Fumaric acid is converted into malic acid in the presence of enzyme fumarase.
9. Formation of oxaloacetic acid: Malic acid is converted into oxaloacetic acid in the presence of enzyme maleate dehydrogenase. This oxaloacetic acid again enters into the cycle and gets converted into acetyl CoA.

Energetics of Citric Acid Cycle

Reactions	ATP molecules formed
1. Pyruvic acid acetyl → CoA	03
2. Isocitric acid → Oxalosuccinate	03
3. α-ketoglutaric acid → Succinyl CoA	03
4. Succinyl CoA → Succinic acid	01
5. Succinic acid → Fumaric acid	02
6. Malic acid → Oxaloacetic acid	03
Total	**15 ATP**

One molecule of glucose gives two molecules of pyruvic acid, therefore, total number of ATP formed in citric acid cycle = 15×2 = 30 ATP

Total number of ATP formed in aerobic oxidation are:
a. From TCA cycle – 30
b. From glucolysis – 08

Total   = 38 ATP

Q 7. Write a note on electron transport chain (ETC/ETS). OR 'Terminal oxidation'. (S. 01, 03; W. 99, 06, 07)

ETS

The process of oxidation of reduced coenzymes ($NADH_2$ and $FADH_2$) and different electron carries through various enzyme systems is called electron transport system or terminal oxidation. In this process the hydrogen from ETS is transferred to molecular oxygen. This is known as terminal oxidation.

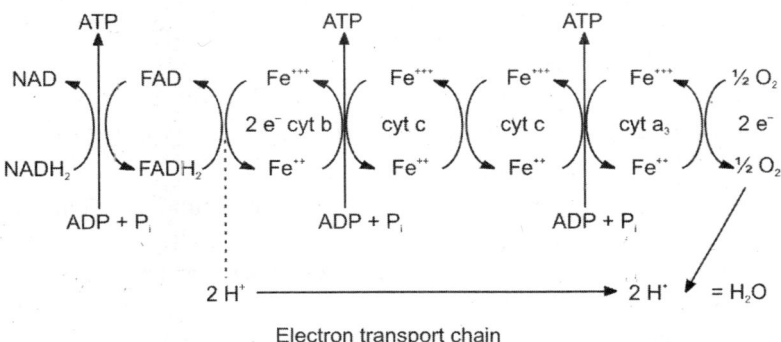

Electron transport chain

Q 8. What is Cori cycle? Explain?

Cori Cycle

The conversion of lactate to glucose takes place entirely in the live⁻ and its re-entry into the muscle, is called Cori cycle.

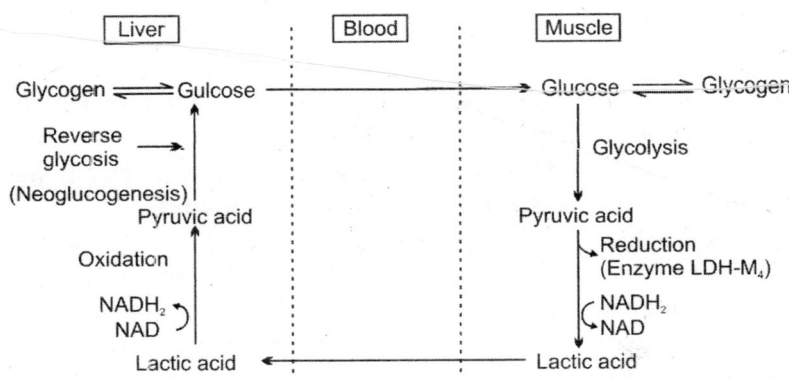

- This cycle is discovered by scientist hence names as Cori cycle.
- It is a cyclic process by which lactic acid is converted into glucose in the liver and after that glucose appears in muscle where glucose can be converted to glycogen and stored in muscles.

- Cori cycle is designed for recycling of lactic acid.
- During vigorous muscular activity, glycogen in muscle is converted in glucose. Then glucose is converted into pyruvic acid by glycolysis.
- Muscles under such condition do not receive sufficient oxygen for normal and complete oxidation of pyruvic acid.
- Now alternatively pyruvic acid is reduced to the lactic acid by enzyme LDH-M_4 and in presence of $NADH_2$ as hydrogen donor. So $NADH_2$ is oxidised to NAD.
- Lactic acid if accumulate in muscles it can result in toxicity, of damaging the muscles so via circulating blood, lactic acid from muscles is taken to liver cells. In the liver cells lactic acid is oxidised to pyruvic acid.
- Finally pyruvic acid is converted into glucose, actually by reverse glycolysis mechanism also called *neoglucogenesis*.
- Glucose thus generated thereafter can be converted to glycogen and stored in liver.
- Whenever necessary glycogen can be converted to glucose again by the action of hormone glucogen. Then glucose via blood stream can be brought to muscles to repeat with same Cori cycle mechanism.

Significance of Cori Cycle

1. It allows proper cycling of lactic acid, so as to avoid toxicity of muscles due to lactic acid accumulations.
2. This mechanism allows skeletal muscles to work without any significant additional supply of oxygen to the muscles.
3. Same mechanism allows conversion of lactic acid to glucose and by proper glucose circulation, it can allow normal operation of energy metabolism in muscles.

Q 9. Write a note on β-oxidation of fatty acids. (S. 96, 97, 01, 02, 03, 04, 05, 06, 07; W. 96, 98, 01, 02, 03, 04, 05, 06, 07)

β-oxidation of Fatty Acids

β-oxidation is a sequential removal of two carbon units as a acetyl-CoA from carboxyl terminal of fatty acids by oxidation.

Reactions of β-oxidation of Fatty Acids

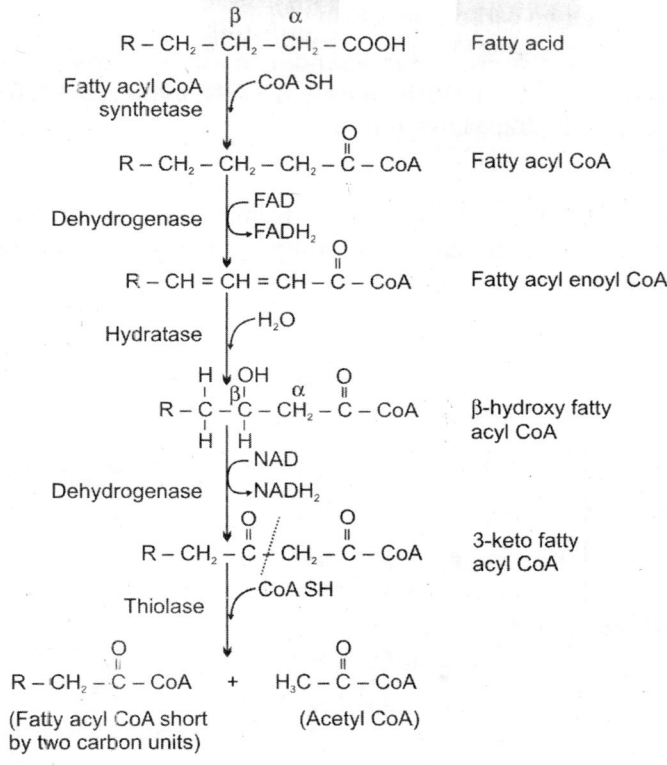

The steps involved in β-oxidation of fatty acids are as follows:

1. *Activation of fatty acid*: In this stage fatty acid gets converted into an active fatty acyl CoA in the presence of fatty acyl CoA synthetase.

2. *Formation of unsaturated acyl CoA*: The hydrogens from fatty acyl CoA are taken up by FAD of the enzymes and thus unsaturated acyl CoA is formed.

3. *Formation of β-hydroxyl acyl CoA*: In this stage one water molecule is added to produce β-hydroxy fatty acyl CoA.

4. *Formation of 3-keto fatty acyl CoA*: The hydrogens from β-hydroxyl acyl CoA are taken up by NAD of the enzyme and thus 3-keto fatty acyl CoA is formed.

5. *Thiolytic cleavage of 3-keto fatty acyl CoA*: 3-keto fatty acyl CoA undergo thiolytic cleavage forms acetyl CoA and active fatty acid containing two carbons less than original.

Q 10. Describe the chemical reactions involved in the formation of urea in the body. OR Write a note on urea cycle. (S. 99, 03, 04, 05, 06, 09; W. 99, 02, 04, 05, 08)

Urea Cycle

Ammonia is combined with CO_2 and forms a urea by various reactions catalysed by the enzymes present in the liver mitochondria through urea cycle.

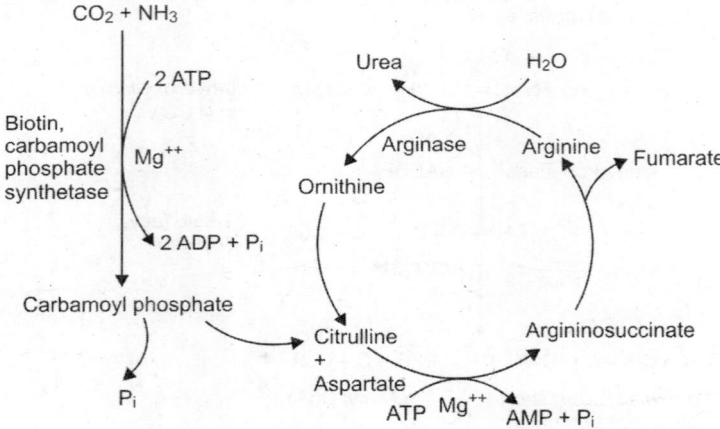

Reactions Involved in Urea Cycle

1. *Formation of carbamoyl phosphate*: Ammonia combines with CO_2 to form carbamoyl phosphate in the presence of biotin and 2 molecules of ATP.
2. *Formation of citrulline*: Citrulline is formed by the transfer of carbamoyl group – $CONH_2$ from carbamoyl to ornithine.
3. *Formation of argininosuccinate*: Amino group of aspartase condenses with citrulline to form argininosuccinate. This reaction is catalysed by argininosuccinate synthetase and requires a molecule of ATP.
4. *Formation of arginine*: Reversible cleavage of argininosuccinate takes place to form arginine and fumarate.
5. *Formation of urea*: It is the last reaction of urea cycle which generates ornithine from arginine for its re-entry in the cycle.

9

Pathology of Blood and Urine

Q 1. Define the terms 'pathology' and 'abnormal urine'.

Pathology (S. 08)

It is the branch of science which deals with the study of diseases and also deals with causes, effects, mechanisms and nature of diseases.

Abnormal Urine/Pathological Urine (S. 09)

The urine which contains abnormal constituents such as sugars, ketone bodies, bile, pus, etc. is known as abnormal urine or pathological urine.

Q 2. What is blood ? Give composition and functions of blood.

Blood (S. 03)

Blood is a fluid connective tissue circulated throughout the body containing blood cells and plasma.

Composition of Blood

Blood is composed of 45% of blood cells and 55% of plasma.

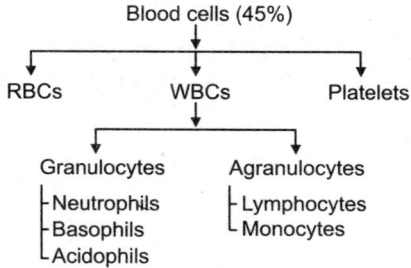

The plasma (55%)
1. *Water*—91 to 92%
2. *Solids* — 8 to 9%

   a. *Inorganic constituents*: Sodium, potassium, calcium.
   b. *Organic constituents*:
      i. Proteins, e.g. albumin, globulin, prothrombin, fibrinogen.
      ii. Non-protein, nitrogenous substances, e.g. neural, uric acid, creatinine.
      iii. Nutrients, e.g. glucose, amino acids, vitamins, glycerol.
      iv. Hormone and enzymes.
      v. Gaseous: O_2, CO_2, nitrogen.
      vi. Antibodies and antitoxins.
      vii. Fats, e.g. neutral fats, phospholipids.
      viii. Colouring matter, e.g. bilirubin.
      ix. Other substances: Internal secretion.

Functions of Blood

1. Blood helps to transport the gases from lungs to the tissues and CO_2 from tissues to the lungs.
2. Blood helps to transport of absorbed digested materials to the tissues of the body.
3. Blood acts as a vehicle through which many substances are transported to their places of activity.
4. Blood helps to drain out waste materials present in the body.
5. Blood acts as a great defensive mechanism.
6. Blood helps to regulate body temperature.
7. Blood maintains acid-base balance.
8. Blood has coagulation property which prevents loss of blood from the body.
9. Blood helps to transport hormones.
10. It regulates to blood pressure.

Q 3. What are lymphocytes? Name two types of lymphocytes. Mention their role in the body (S. 98; W. 96, 97, 04)

Lymphocytes are granular leukocytes, i.e. WBCs. The normal count of lymphocyte is 25 to 30% of total WBCs. Lymphocytes are made in lymph nodes and in the lymphatic tissue which is present in spleen, liver and bone marrow. There are two types of lymphocytes.

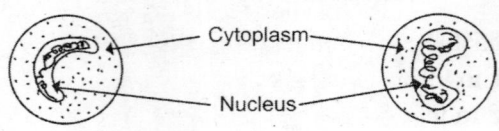

a. Small lymphocytes (T-cells), (b) Large lymphocytes (B-cells)

The large lymphocytes are considered to the younger forms of small lymphocytes. They are found to contain abundant cytoplasm which stains, pale-blue and non-granular. The nucleus is very large, single, generally spherical and stains blue. The small lymphocytes ranges from 7 to 10 μ in size and large up to 20 μ.

Functions

   i. They are responsible from formation of antibodies.

   ii. They manufactures β and γ serum globulins.

  iii. They plays important role in defensive mechanism.

  iv. They helps in repairment of inflamed tissues.

   v. The small lymphocytes have very long life span and play an important role in immunity.

Q 4. What are leukocytes? Give different types of leukocytes. (S. 02, 03, 07; W. 05)

The leukocytes are colourless cells containing, irregular shaped large nucleus and are named as white blood cells.

The normal count of leukocytes is 6000 to 10,000/mm^3 of blood. On the basis of granules, leukocytes are classified into two groups.

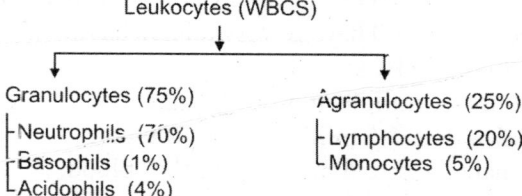

A. Granulocytes

They constitute about 75%. These cells contains granules in the cytoplasm hence called granulocytes.

1. *Neutrophils*: The granules of these cells are stained by neutral dye. The nucleus is many lobed.
   - *Functions:* They ingest the microbes and destroy it by phagocytosis.
2. *Basophils*: The granules of these cells are stained by basic dye. The nucleus is usually oval or slightly kidney shaped.
   - *Functions:* They are responsible for destruction of products of antigen-antibody reactions.

3. *Eosinophils*: The granules of these cells are stained by red acidic dye called as eosinophil. The nucleus is many lobed.
   - *Function:* Phagocytosis.

B. Agranulocytes

These are mononuclear cells and they do not show presence of granules in their cytoplasm.
1. *Monocytes*: These are large cells with large nucleus. The nucleus is convoluted kidney shaped.
   - *Function*: They gives phagocytic action.
2. *Lymphocytes*: These are produced in the lymph glands hence called as lymphocytes.
   - i *Small lymphocytes*: The nucleus is thin rim around the nucleus and stained by basic stains.
   - ii. *Large lymphocytes*: The nucleus is oval rounded or kidney shaped and is stained by basic stains.
   - *Functions*: They are responsible for the development of immunity against foreign substances such as microorganisms.

Q 5. What are erythrocytes? Explain (RBCs). (S. 98; W. 01)

These are small, circular, disc shaped cells suspended in blood plasma. All the cells in group appears as a red in colour and thus the blood becomes a red coloured. They are very minute having diameter 7.2 μ.

Normal values of RBCs:
- i. In adult—5 millions/mm^3 of blood
- ii. In male—5 to 5.5 millions/mm^3 of blood
- iii. In female—4.5 to 5 millions/mm^3 of blood.

RBCs are produced in the red bone marrow. The process of formation of RBCs in the blood is called erythropoieses.

The RBCs contain a substance known as haemoglobin and is enclosed in the stroma of RBCs.

Haemoglobin is a complex protein of high molecular weight. It consists of a protein material called as globin and nonprotein material called as 'haem'. The haem contains iron which gives red colour to the haemoglobin.

Total life span of RBCs is 120 days.

Functions of RBCs/Erythrocytes

1. It transports the gases such as O$_2$ and CO$_2$ in the form of oxyhaemoglobin and carboxyhaemoglobin.

2. It maintains acid–base balance by buffering action of haemoglobin.
3. RBCs helps to maintain viscosity of blood.
4. RBCs maintain iron balance of the body.
5. Various pigments are derived from haemoglobin after disintegration of RBCs, e.g. bilirubin and biliverdin.

Q 6. What are platelets? Give their importance. (S. 02; W. 08)

- Platelet is also known as thrombocyte.
- These are minute spherical structures present in the blood.
- They are produced by large cell, i.e. megakaryotes present in the bone marrow.
- They are disc-shaped, non-nucleated bodies about 2–4 µ in diameter.
- The average life span of platelet is about 5 to 10 days and are destroyed in the spleen.
- The normal count of platelet is 3 to 4 lacs/mm^3 of blood.
- The platelet contains thrombokinase or thromboplastin which is liberated when platelet comes in contact with rough surface and it plays an important role in clotting of blood.

Functions of Platelets

1. The platelets contains thromboplastin which plays an important role in blood clotting.
2. The platelet agglutination helps in the control of bleeding as they seal the small leakings of injured blood vessels or capillaries.
3. The platelets acts as protective measure for endothelial lining of blood vessels.
4. The platelets releases histamine and 5-hydroxy-tryptamine to induce vasoconstriction.

Q 7. Explain the terms.

a. *Purpura* (*W. 04*): It is the abnormal condition of blood in which platelet count is below normal:
   - *Symptoms:*
     i. Red patches beneath the skin.
     ii. Bleeding in the skin and mucous membrane.
     iii. The appearance of lesions.
     iv. The colour of lesion is first red and the fading to a brownish yellow.

    v. The clotting time remains normal but bleeding time is pro-
longed.

b. *Thrombocytopenia*: A decrease in the platelet count below 70,000/
mm^3 of blood produces increased tendency to capillary bleeding.
This condition is called thrombocytopenia.

Q 8. Give the composition of normal urine (physiological urine). (W. 98, 99, 01, 08)

Composition of Urine

Water	96%	
Urea	2%	
Uric acid	Chlorides	
Creatinine	Phosphates	
Ammonia	Sulphates	
Sodium	Oxalates	2%
Potassium	Glucose	
Hippuric acid	Oxalic acid	

Characteristic of Urine

1. Urine is amber in colour
2. Specific gravity is 1.020 to 1.030
3. Acidic in nature
4. Healthy adult passes 1000 to 1500 ml of urine per day.

Q 9. What are the abnormal constituents of urine? Give their significance in disease or pathological conditions. (S. 96, 97, 98, 00, 01, 02, 03, 04, 05, 07; W. 97, 98, 99, 02, 03, 04, 05, 06)

The following are abnormal constituents of urine.

Abnormal constituents	Significance disease
1. Proteins	Proteinuria
2. Sugar	Glycosuria
3. Ketone bodies	Ketonuria
4. Bile pigments and salts	Jaundice
5. Blood	Haematuria
6. Pus	Pyuria

1. *Protein:* The presence of proteins in the urine is called proteinuria.
The presence of albumin and globulin in urine is called albumin-
uria and globulinuria.

The proteinuria results in following pathological conditions:
  i. Nephritis
  ii. Nephrotic syndrome
  iii. Renal tuberculosis
  iv. Bacterial infections in kidney
  v. Mercury poisoning
  vi. Proteinuria is observed in severe exercise, high protein meal, pregnancy, etc.

2. *Sugars*: The presence of sugar in urine is described as glycosuria. This is associated with the increased blood sugar levels exceeding the threshold level. The glycosuria occurs in the following pathological conditions:
  i. Diabetes mellitus
  ii. Renal glycosuria.

3. *Ketone bodies* (*acetone bodies*): Under certain conditions of the body, carbohydrates utilization is not up to the required quantity, the increased quantity of fats are broken down for the production of energy.

   This results in the formation of ketone bodies which appears in the blood called as **ketonemia** and the excretion of the ketone bodies in the urine is called **ketonuria**.

   Thus ketosis is a process in which ketonemia and ketonuria occurs. The *acetone, acetoacetic acid,* and β-hydroxy butyric acid are collectively described as ketone bodies.

   Ketonuria is found in the following pathological conditions:
  i. Carbohydrate starvation.
  ii. Pregnancy
  iii. In anaesthesia.

4. *Bile pigments and salts*: Sodium glycolate and sodium taurocholate are bile salts while bilirubin and biliverdin are bile pigments. The presence of bile pigments and bile salts produces greenish yellow, greenish brown colour to the urine.

   In defective liver function and when the bile passage is obstructive then bile appears in the urine.

   Bile pigments appears in all types of jaundice.
  i. Haemolytic jaundice
  ii. Obstructive jaundice
  iii. Toxic jaundice.

5. *Blood*: When blood appears in urine the condition is called haematuria. In haemoglobinuria, the only haemoglobin pigment is found in urine.

   • *Pathological conditions*:
     i. Haematuria occurs due to kidney lesions.
     ii. Hemoglobinuria occurs in enteric fever, malaria, haemolytic poisoning.
     iii. Snake venom causes haemolysis which results in presence of haemoglobin in urine.

6. *Pus*: Presence of pus in the urine is termed as pyuria.

   Pyuria is caused due to inflammation of the urinary bladder, urethra and pelvis of kidney.

Q 10. Write a note on 'megaloblastic anaemia'. (S. 96, 97, 99, 01, 02, 04; W. 97, 00, 02, 06, 07)

It is also known as macrocytic anaemia.

It occurs due to stopped development of erythrocyte at megaloblastic stage. It is because of deficiency of vitamin B_{12} and folic acid.

It characterised by large red cells than normal.

The life span of these cells is also reduced.

The average red cell size is greater than normal, hence it is termed as macrocytic anemia.

The deficiency of vitamin B_{12} is the result of absence of 'intrinsic factor' from the gastric secretion.

• *Main characters of this anaemia are:*
   i. Much large RBCs than normal
   ii. Presence of large and pale nucleus in RBC
   iii. Immature RBCs appear in blood circulation due to decrease in physiology.

• *Symptoms:*
   i. RBCs of different size, shape and colour.
   ii. RBCs with large and pale nucleus.
   iii. Polychromatic pigment granules in RBCs.
   iv. General nervousness.
   v. Sensations such as numbness and tingling.
   vi. Occurrence of pins and needles in the finger and toes.
   vii. Very reduced RBC count.
   viii. Decreased O_2 carrying capacity.

- *Treatment*:
    i. Increased dietary intake of vitamin B_{12} or vitamin B_{12} tablets as therapeutic treatment.
    ii. Intramuscular injection of vitamin B_{12}.

Q 11. Write a note on "sickle cell anaemia". (S. 96, 97, 99, 01, 02, 05, 06; W. 97, 00, 02, 06, 07)

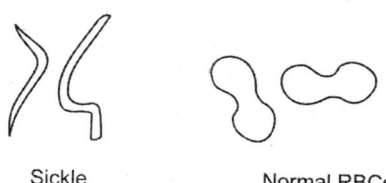

Sickle   Normal RBCs

Sickle cell anaemia is also called sickle cell disease. In this anaemia there is abnormal formation of RBC and they are having a sickle type.

The main reason of this anaemia is the bone marrow produce abnormal type of haemoglobin. It is a haemoglobin of "S" type instead of normal haemoglobin "A". The difference between two is a small change in structure of molecule.

Haemoglobin "S" is peculiar sensitive to a lowered oxygen supply.

Red cells with this type of haemoglobin form sickle or cresent shapes when subjected to lower doxygen concentration. The sickle cells do not pass through the small blood capillaries readily and hence may block the blood supply to vital organs. Patient with sickle cell disease show a marked susceptibility to infections.

- *Characteristic/symptoms of sickle cell anaemia*:
    i. Sickle shaped RBCs (observed under microscope).
    ii. Sudden, severe abdominal pains followed by excretion of dark urine.
    iii. Blockage of blood capillaries may block the blood supply to vital organs.
    iv. Decreased blood supply and decreased O_2 supply to body organs.
    v. General tissue damage due to local necrosis.
- *Treatments*:
    i. The sickle cell patient should avoid situations where a lowered concentration of oxygen may be present.

ii. Reaching high attitudes and air polluted areas should be avoided.

iii. Patient should obtain prompt medical care in case of cold pneumonia.

Q 12. Write a note on "microcytic anaemia". (S. 00, 01)

- This is also called iron deficiency anaemia because, the deficiency of iron causes the bone marrow to produce small red blood cells.
- RBCs are pale and less in numbers.
- Such anaemia is common in women than in men and it is found common in Indian women.
- The main cause of this anaemia is iron deficiency followed by bone marrow depression.
- The iron deficiency may be due to:
  i. Dietary deficiency of iron
  ii. Hookworm infestation
  iii. Lack of HCl in stomach, where HCl is required for normal absorption of iron.
- *Symptoms*:
  i. Abnormally small sized RBCs containing very low haemoglobin
  ii. RBCs of very pale colour
  iii. Shortness of breath with exercise
  iv. Faintness
  v. Headache
  vi. Total RBC count is very low
  vii. Pale colour of skin and nails.
- *Treatments*:
  i. Iron therapy through proper diet
  ii. Actually proper cause of iron deficiency is found out and patient is treated accordingly
  iii. Antiworm drugs should be used to kill the hookworms.

Q 13. Write a note on "haemolytic anaemia".

It is the condition of abnormal destruction of RBCs in blood called haemolysis. Such destruction may occur in blood stream.

- *Causes/Reasons:*
  i. Poisoning by various substances like lead, mercury, arsenic, etc.

ii. Toxins produced by bacteria called *Streptococcus haemolyticus.*

iii. Infection by malarial parasite as *Plasmodium species.*

iv. RBC destruction due to cancer or malignancy.

v. Mismatching of blood groups due to incompatible blood transfusion.

- *Symptoms*:
    i. Decreased RBC count
    ii. Decreased haemoglobin content
    iii. Low O_2 carrying capacity
    iv. Breathlessness
    v. Restlessness
    vi. Very pale skin.

- *Treatments*:
    i. Proper blood transfusion to compensate RBC loss is main treatment
    ii. Antidote in case of poisoning
    iii. Antimalarial drug treatment in case of malaria
    iv. Avoiding blood group mismatching during transfusion
    v. Preventing measures for streptococcal infection.

Q 14. Write a note on "haemorrhagic anaemia".

Haemorrhage means blood loss due to any reason, so can result in condition called haemorrhagic anaemia.

- *Causes/Reasons*
    i. Peptic ulcer of severe bleeding to blood vomits.
    ii. Intestinal ulcers of severe degree leading to blood loss through stools.
    iii. Dysmenorrhoea is abnormally heavy bleeding during menstruation in women.
    iv. Heavy bleeding wounds in case of accident victim.
    v. Blood vomits as in case of blood cancer, etc.

- *Symptoms*:
    i. Low blood volume
    ii. Low RBC count
    iii. Reduced haemoglobin content of blood
    iv. Pale skin and nails
    v. General fatigue
    vi. Faintness.

- *Treatments*:
  - i. Stop the bleeding immediately.
  - ii. Earliest blood transfusion to compensate blood loss is another treatment.
  - iii. Treating the patient specifically by finding actual cause of bleeding.
  - iv. Symptomatic treatment can be conducted.

Q 15. Explain the terms.

1. *Anaemia (S. 07, 08, 09; W. 05)*: Anaemia means reduction in amount of oxygen carrying capacity of blood, i.e. haemoglobin. Deficiency of RBCs causes anaemia.
   - *Causes/reasons of anaemia*:
     - i. Due to excessive blood loss, i.e. severe haemorrhage.
     - ii. Failure of function of red bone marrow so that no blood cells are formed.
     - iii. Due to increased destruction of RBCs by haemolysis.
     - iv. Defective formation of RBCs includes abnormal reduction of RBCs in the blood.
     - v. Dietary deficiency of iron may cause decrease in % of RBC causing anaemia.
   - *Type of anaemia*:
     - i. Megaloblastic anaemia
     - ii. Sickle cell anaemia
     - iii. Pernicious anaemia
     - iv. Haemolytic anaemia
     - v. Haemorrhagic anaemia
     - vi. Iron deficiency anaemia
     - vii. Hypochromic anaemia
     - viii. Hypoplastic anaemia
     - ix. Nutritional anaemia.
   - *Treatments of anaemia*:
     - i. Increase dietary intake of vitamin B_{12}
     - ii. Use of haematinics
     - iii. Iron therapy through proper diet
     - iv. To prevent blood loss due to any reason
     - v. Blood transfusion to compensate blood loss or RBCs.

2. *Polycythaemia (S. 08)*: An abnormal increase in RBCs in the blood is called as polycythaemia.

   Due to increase in erythrocyte, the viscosity of blood increases and rate of blood flow becomes and increases risk of intravascular clotting (thrombosis). This also increases BP.
   - *Types of polycythaemia*
     i. *Primary polycythaemia*: In this case along with increased number of red cells, the bone marrow is markedly hyperplastic. Thus skin and mucous membranes of the mouth are red. The conjunctiva is also red.
     ii. *Secondary polycythaemia*: In this case there is a large increase in red cells in the condition of insufficient oxygenation.

3. *Leukaemia (increased in WBCs)*: It is malignant disease of bone marrow that results in uncontrolled increase in production of leukocytes in blood. Immature forms of WBCs make their appearance in the circulating blood in leukaemia condition. It is also called as cancer of blood.
   - *Causes of leukaemia*:
     i. Ionising radiations produced by X-ray or radioactive isotopes are known to cause malignant changes in the precursors of WBCs. The genetic material of the cells is changed. Some cells die while others reproduce at abnormally rapid rate.
     ii. Some chemicals used in general or work environments are known to change the genetic make up of WBC precursor in the bone marrow.

4. *Lecopenia (decrease in WBCs)*: This is the condition in which there is a decrease in WBC count below 4000/mm^3 of blood. Commonly this disease is caused due to fall in the count of neutrophil cells.

5. *Leucocytosis*: It is the abnormal condition in which there is an increased number of WBCs in the blood above normal range. It is observed in the some respiratory diseases like allergic bronchitis.

6. *Granulocytosis*: This is the pathological condition indicated by presence of increased number of granulocytes in blood.

7. *Agranulocytosis*: It is the condition of complete absence of granulocytes from blood or bone marrow.

Different reasons can lead to such condition, e.g. suppression of the function of bone marrow.

Agranulocytosis can often resulting in high fever, weakness, and ulceration of the mucous membrane.

8. *Haemophilia (bleeding disease)*: This is a hereditary disease which runs in families. In this condition the bleeding occurs continuously by even a small skin cut or puncture.

A person suffering from haemophilia can lead to death while even small injury or small cut, as the blood lacks the ability to clot. A person suffering from this disease is known as haemophilic person.

In this hereditary disorder the female is carried while effect is pronounced in male.

9. *Eosinophilia*: It is abnormal condition indicated by increased in number of eosinophils in blood, e.g. eosinophils increases in the conditions like malaria, dengue and in case of treatment of antibiotics.

10. *Erythrocytopaenia*: It is the pathological condition of decreased number of RBCs in peripheral blood vessels.

11. *Erythrocytosis*: It is the condition indicated by presence of increased RBC count much above normal and it is associated with increase in total blood volume.

Q 16. What are ketone bodies/acetone bodies? How are ketone bodies detected in urine? (S. 02; W. 98, 00, 01)

- Acetone, acetoacetic acid, β-hydroxy butyric acid are collectively described as ketone bodies.
- Only 3–15 mg of ketone bodies are excreted in urine normally.
- The increased amount of ketone bodies are excreted in urine in starvation, diabetes mellitus, pregnancy, ether anaesthesia.
- Ketone bodies in urine detected by following tests.

1. *Rothera's test*:
   - *Principle*: Acetoacetic acid forms a complex with sodium nitroprusside in alkaline solution developing a purple colour.
   - *Test*:
     i. Saturate 5 ml of urine with solid ammonium sulphate by shaking it vigorously.

ii. Then add 2 drops of freshly prepared 5% solution of sodium nitroprusside and 1 ml of ammonium hydroxide.

iii. Allow to stand for a while.

iv. A permanganate or purple colour develops just above the layer of ammonium sulphate indicates the presence of acetone bodies.

2. *Gerhardt tests*:
   - *Principle*: Acetoacetic acid gives a red colour with $FeCl_3$.
   - *Test*:

     i. Add 5% ferric chloride solution drop by drop to about 5 ml urine till no more precipitate of ferric chloride is formed.

     ii. Filter and to the filtrate add some more ferric chloride solution.

     iii. The development of red colour indicates the presence of acetoacetic acid.

Q 17. How albumin (protein) is detected in urine?

Abnormal albumin in urine is detected by:

1. *Sulphosalicylic acid test*: Albumin is denatured by sulphosalicylic acid causing coagulation.
   - *Test*: Add a few drops of sulphosalicylic acid to 2 ml of clear urine. A turbidity indicates presence of albumin.

2. *Heller's nitric acid ring rest*: Nitric acid causes the precipitation of proteins.
   - *Test:*

     i. To 3 ml of nitric acid in a marrow tube add 3 ml of urine in such a way that the two liquids do not mix.

     ii. The presence of white ring at the function of two fluids indicates the presence of albumin.

Q 18. How bile salts and bile pigments are detected in urine? (S. 97, 03; W. 99)

1. *Bile salts*: Sodium glycocholate and sodium taurocholate are the bile salts, found in urine in defective liver function and is the characteristic of the jaundice.

   Hay's test for bile pigments: Bile salts reduces the surface tension present in the urine for which the sulphur powder sinks.

- *Test*:
    i. Fill half of a test tube with urine and another test tube with water.
    ii. Sprinkle gently same sulphur powder on the surface of two liquors.
    iii. The sulphur powder spontaneously sinks in the test tube containing urine which indicates presence of bile salts.
    iv. But in other test tube containing water, sulphur powder does not sink.

2. *Bile pigments*: Bilirubin and biliverdin are the bile pigments. Bile pigments are detected by Fouchet's test.

   Fauchet's test
   - *Principle*: Bilirubin is precipitated by barium chloride. This bilirubin is oxidised to green biliverdin by Fouchet's reagent.
   - *Test* (*Fauchet's test*)
       i. Acidify 10 ml of urine with a few drops of dilute acetic acid and add 5 ml of 10% solution.
       ii. If there is no much precipitate add 2 drops of saturated solution so magnesium sulphate, mix and allow to stand for few minutes.
       iii. Filter and unfold the filter paper.
       iv. Add one drop of Fouchet's reagent to precipitate.
       v. The development of green colouration indicates the presence of bile pigments.

Q 19. How sugar is detected in urine? (S. 03)

Sugar is detected in urine by:
a. Benedict's test
b. Fehling's test

a. Benedict's Test

  i. Add 0.5 ml of urine to about 5 ml of Benedict qualitative reagent.
 ii. Boil it for 2 minutes by holding the test tube firmly with a test tube holder.
iii. A light green, yellow and brick red precipitate indicates the presence of reducing sugar in urine.
 iv. The various coloured precipitates depends on the concentration of reducing sugar in urine which give rough estimation of concentration, as follows:

Light green precipitate	0.1 to 0.5% of sugar
Green precipitate	0.1 to 1% of sugar
Yellow precipitate	1 to 2% of sugar
Brick red precipitate	Above 2% of sugar

b. Fehling's Test

Boil sugar solution and Fehling's solution for two minutes gives formation of brick red precipitate which indicates the reducing sugar.

Q 20. Discuss bile salts and bile pigments. In which disease these appear in urine? (S. 96; W. 99)

- *Bile salts*: Sodium glycocholate and sodium taurocholate are bile salts which acts as emulsifying agent and emulsify fats. They activate pancreatic lipase and cholesterol esterase.
- *Bile pigments*: Bilirubin and biliverdin are the bile pigments formed from the breakdown of haemoglobin. Bile pigments are excreted in bile.
- In obstructive jaundice, bile salts and bile pigments appears in urine.

Board Question Papers

(From Summer 1996 to Summer 2017)

Summer Examination 1996
D Pharm First Year
Biochemistry and Clinical Pathology

Q 1. Attempt any _five_ of the following:

   a. Define:

      i. Mutarotation   ii. Reducing sugars

   b. Draw the structure of:

      i. D-glucose   ii. D-fructose

   c. What happens to the body when excess vitamin A is consumed?

   d. Explain the term "unit of enzyme activity".

   e. Define:

      i. Saponification number   ii. Iodine number

   f. Name the major sites where glycogen is stored.

   g. Name the essential amino acids.

Q 2. Attempt any _four_ of the following:

   a. Define and classify proteins giving suitable examples.

   b. Give the principles of following qualitative tests of carbohydrates:

      i. Molisch's test   ii. Benedict's test

   c. Discuss in brief the role of lipids.

   d. Explain the role of vitamin A in vision.

   e. Write short note on role of calcium in life processes.

   f. Describe the role played by cell nucleus.

Q 3. Attempt any _four_ of the following:

   a. Discuss in brief concept of enzymic action.

   b. Explain "TCA cycle".

   c. Define anaemia. What is megaloblastic anaemia?

   d. Discuss the primary structure of proteins.

e. Define and classify carbohydrates giving suitable examples.

f. Write a note on acid-base behaviours of amino acids.

Q 4. Attempt any *four* of the following:

a. What are coenzymes? Illustrate with examples.

b. Explain water balance of a body.

c. What are the diseases which occur due to disorders of lipid metabolism?

d. Mention different factors affecting enzyme catalysed reaction. What is the effect of temperature on it?

e. How lipids are digested in the body?

f. How are amino acids detected? Give the use of ninhydrin for detection.

Q 5. Attempt any *four* of the following:

a. What are abnormal constituents of urine? Give their significance in diseases.

b. Explain following qualitative tests of amino acids.
   i. Xanthoproteic test   ii. Million's test

c. Give the properties, structure and uses of sucrose.

d. What are essential fatty acids? Discuss with examples.

e. Define and classify vitamins giving suitable examples. Give the biochemical role of folic acid.

f. Explain the formation of urea in the body.

Q 6. Attempt any *four* of the following:

a. Give the major functions of minerals in life processes.

b. Give the therapeutic and pharmaceutical importance of enzyme.

c. Explain the term "abnormal metabolism". Illustrate with examples.

d. Discuss bile salts and bile pigments. In which disease these appear in urine?

e. What is phenyl ketonuria and alkaptonuria? Explain.

f. Explain beta-oxidation of fatty acids.

Winter Examination 1996
D Pharm First Year
Biochemistry and Clinical Pathology

Q 1. Attempt any *five* of the following:

a. Define the following terms:
   i. Coenzyme   ii. Co-factor

b. Mention the different qualitative tests for proteins.

    c. Draw the structure of maltose.

    d. Explain the term 'rancidity'.

    e. Explain the term 'catabolism'.

    f. Mention different types of anaemias.

    g. Write names of aromatic amino acids.

Q 2. Attempt any *four* of the following:

    a. Define and classify amino acids giving suitable examples.

    b. Discuss the biological value of proteins.

    c. Write short note on protein deficiency diseases.

    d. Describe the role of carbohydrates.

    e. Give significance of following qualitative tests of carbohydrates.

        i. Fehling's test   iii. Seliwanoff's test

        ii. Barfoed's test

    f. Describe the role of mitochondria in the cell.

Q 3. Attempt any *four* of the following:

    a. Give the properties, structure and uses of lactose.

    b. What are lipids? Classify with suitable examples.

    c. Mention chemical constants for fats. Explain iodine number.

    d. Name the respective vitamin, nutritional deficiency of which leads to:

        i. Xerophthalmia   v. Pernicious anaemia

        ii. Rickets   vi. Blood clotting disorder

        iii. Pellagra   vii. Beriberi

        iv. Scurvy

    e. Give the qualitative tests for lipids.

    f. Write a note on mutarotation.

Q 4. Attempt any *four* of the following:

    a. Give the absorption, excretion and functions of vitamin D.

    b. Explain the biochemical role of pyridoxal phosphate.

    c. Explain the role of sodium in life processes.

    d. Mention various factors which affect the enzyme catalysed reaction. Discuss the effect of enzyme concentration on it.

    e. Describe the role of water in life processes.

    f. Write a note on amino acid catabolism.

Q 5. Attempt any *four* of the following:

    a. Mention the important minerals present in the body. Give the functions of iron in life processes.

    b. Give the biochemical role of thiamine.

    c. Define inhibition. Give its different types. Explain competitive inhibition.

    d. What do you understand by the term phenyl ketonuria? Explain it.

    e. Write short note on glycolysis.

    f. Name the diseases related to carbohydrate metabolism and explain in detail any one of them.

Q 6. Attempt any *four* of the following:

    a. Give the therapeutic importance of enzymes.

    b. Explain the biochemical process 'β-oxidation' of fatty acids.

    c. Give the role of lymphocytes and platelets in health and diseases.

    d. Explain the following terms:

        i. Polycythemia   iii. Ketosis

        ii. Glycosuria

    e. Write short note on polypeptides.

    f. Write a note on abnormal metabolism.

Summer Examination 1997
D Pharm First Year
Biochemistry and Clinical Pathology

Q 1. Attempt in brief any *four*:

    a. What do you mean by the term "metabolism" and give its importance in a living cell.

    b. Define "vitamins" and classify them with one example.

    c. What are carbohydrates and give its classification.

    d. Explain the role of phospholipids in biological membrane.

    e. Define 'enzymes'. Give their major classification.

    f. Give the importance of minerals in a biological system.

Q 2. Give the biochemical role of any *four*:

    a. Thiamine

    b. Iron

    c. Calcium

    d. Pyridoxine

    e. Magnesium

Q 3. Write short notes on any *four*:

    a. Competitive inhibition

    b. Ozasone formation

    c. Mutarotation

    d. Reducing sugars

    e. Lymphocytes

    f. Sickle-cell anaemia

Q 4. Solve any *four* of the following:

a. Discuss in brief how bile salts and bile pigments and detected in urine.

b. Give the principle involved in:
   i. Molisch's test   ii. Million's test

c. Explain with chemical reaction "enediol formation" in monosaccharides.

d. Define:
   i. Biochemistry   ii. Cell

e. Name the diseases related with carbohydrate metabolism.

f. Write short note on "glycosuria".

Q 5. Explain the following biochemical processes of any *four*:

a. Glycolysis

b. Beta-oxidation

c. Ornithine cycle

d. Transamination

e. Ketone bodies

f. Deamination

Q 6. Solve any *four* of the following:

a. Define "protein" and give diseases related with its metabolism.

b. Define "anomers" and "epimer" with suitable example.

c. Name any four essential "amino acids" and draw structure of serine.

d. Give the action of acid on monosaccharides with reaction.

e. Explain in brief about cholesterol and diseases related with cholesterol.

f. Give any four normal and abnormal constituents of urine.

Winter Examination 1997
D Pharm First Year
Biochemistry and Clinical Pathology

Q 1. Attempt any *five* bits. Each bits carries equal marks:

a. Explain the term rancidification of fats.

b. Define and explain the formation of peptide and polypeptides bond.

c. Define and explain the terms iodine number and formation of glycerol tristearate.

d. Give the structure of stearic acid, oleic acid and linoleic acid.

e. What is the disease—rickets and beriberi. What are their causes?

f. Explain the alkaline hydrolysis of fats and oils.

Q 2. Attempt any *two* bits:
   a. State the classification, general formula and structure of α-amino acids.
   b. Explain the biological function of proteins. State their importance in growth of animal and plants.
   c. Explain the primary and secondary structure of protein.
   d. How the protein reacts with the following reagents:
      i. Xanthoprotein test   iii. Nitroprusside reagent
      ii. Ninhydrin reagent

Q 3. Attempt any *three* bits:
   a. What are the fats and oils? Differentiate between them.
   b. How many kinds of phospholipids are there? Give the function and structure of sphingomyelins.
   c. What important role the lipids play in the growth of our body?
   d. Describe the biochemical role of minerals iron and sodium in our body.
   e. State the properties of water. Why it is important in body metabolism?

Q 4. Attempt any *three* bits:
   a. What different products are obtain upon oxidation and reduction of α D?
   b. Give the structure of sucrose and maltose and fructose.
   c. Give the identification test for monosaccharides and disccharides sugar.
   d. What are the abnormal constituents of urine? Give their significance in disease.
   e. What is megaloblastic anaemia? How it is treated?

Q 5. Attempt any *three* bits:
   a. Illustrate the biochemical role of vitamin D. State what role it plays in calcium metabolism.
   b. State the role and structure of vitamin riboflavin (vitamin B_2) and bioline (vitamin H).
   c. Explain the following terms:
      i. Rickets   iii. Egg white injury
      ii. Beriberi
   d. Write notes on:
      i. K_m and V_{max}
      ii. Metal coenzymes
      iii. Optimum pH for enzyme action

Q 6. Attempt any *two* bits:
a. Describe the various characteristics of proteins.
b. Discuss the biological importance of glycogen.
c. What is ATP? Give its role in biological system?
d. Write notes on:
    i. Insulin   ii. Maple syrup disease

Summer Examination 1998
D Pharm First Year
Biochemistry and Clinical Pathology

Q 1. Attempt any *five* of the following:
a. Draw the structure of sucrose.
b. Define isoenzyme with example.
c. Give the symptoms of beriberi.
d. Define:
    i. Acetyl value
    ii. Acid value
e. Explain the following terms:
    i. Glycogenesis
    ii. Glycogenolysis.
f. What is active site of enzyme?
g. Enumerate various factors that affect enzyme activities.

Q 2. Attempt any *four* of the following:
a. Give the significance of precipitation reactions of proteins. Explain biuret test.
b. What are three main features of amino acids? Give essential amino acids.
c. Give the osazone test of carbohydrates.
d. Give the significance of various chemical constants for fats.
e. Describe the biochemical role of folic acid.
f. Describe various parts of cell.

Q 3. Attempt any *four* of the following:
a. Give properties, structure and uses of maltose.
b. How do you classify lipids?
c. Give the functions and deficiency diseases of vitamin 'C'.
d. Explain the following terms:
    i. Rickets
    ii. Pellagra

e. What are lipids? Explain the role of phospholipids in biological membrane.

f. Write a note on medicinal importance of enzymes.

Q 4. Attempt any *four* of the following:

a. Give the biochemical role of vitamin B_2.

b. Write the major functions of phosphorus.

c. Describe the water balance of our body.

d. What are trace elements? Give the biochemical role of copper in the body.

e. Define enzymes. Give their classification.

f. What are coenzymes? Describe coenzymic role of nicotinamide adenine dinucleotide.

Q 5. Attempt any *four* of the following:

a. What is the effect of following factors on enzyme catalysed reaction:
   i. pH
   ii. Presence of activators

b. Describe the abnormal metabolism of lipids with reference to ketone body formation.

c. Discuss the mechanism of enzyme action.

d. What is transamination? How it differs from deamination?

e. Describe Krebs cycle giving reactions involved.

f. What are the functions of electrolytes in life processes.

Q 6. Attempt any *four* of the following:

a. Describe abnormal erythrocytic cells and their significance.

b.   i. Define pathological urine
   ii. Match the following:

Abnormal constituents	Disease of urine
1. Sugar	i. Jaundice
2. Albumin	ii. Diabetes mellitus
3. Bile pigments	iii. Nephritis
	iv. Define polyuria.

c. What are lymphocytes? Describe their role in health and diseases.

d. Write a note on abnormal metabolism of protein.

e. Answer the following:
   i. Define polypeptides. Give one example of polypeptides which act as hormone.
   ii. Give the name of antioxidant of fat soluble vitamin.
   iii. Which is the major element present in extracellular fluid?

f. Give the classification of carbohydrates.

Winter Examination 1998
D Pharm First Year
Biochemistry and Clinical Pathology

Q 1.

a. **Select best answer:**
   i. Sulphur containing amino acid is:
      1. Arginine
      2. Lysine
      3. Serine
      4. Methionine
   ii. Deficiency of niacin causes:
      1. Scurvy
      2. Pellagra
      3. Nyctalopia
      4. Rickets
   iii. Essential fatty acid is:
      1. Stearic acid
      2. Palmitic acid
      3. Lauric acid
      4. Linoleic acid
   iv. One of the important steroid is:
      1. Tryptophan
      2. Fatty acids
      3. Cholesterol
      4. Piperidine
   v. Phosphorylation of the metabolite is carried out by kinases in the presence of:
      1. Acetyl coenzyme A
      2. Ascorbic acid
      3. Pyruvic acid
      4. ATP

b. **Fill in the blanks (any *five*):**
   i. The high blood level of _____ in blood is called galactosuria.
   ii. Deficiency of vitamin C, produces _____.
   iii. Carbohydrates that differ in the configuration around carbonyl carbon atom is called _____.
   iv. Breakdown of larger molecules with the release of energy is called _____.
   v. The coenzyme forms of riboflavin are FAD and _____.
   vi. The presence of blood in urine is called _____.

Q 2. Solve any *four* of the following:

a. How carbohydrates are classified on chemical basis?

b. Give any *two* identification tests for reducing sugars.

c. How do waxes differ from fats? How do fats and oils differs from each other?

d. Name *two* colour tests for cholesterol. Give the structure of cholesterol.

e. Describe in brief classification of proteins.

f. Explain acid-base behaviour of amino acids.

Q 3. Solve any *four* of the following:

   a. Write short note on competitive inhibition by giving suitable examples.

   b. Explain the following terms:

      i. Prosthetic group   ii. Metalloenzymes

   c. What do you understand by specificity of enzymes? Mention the various kinds of specificities observed in different enzymic reactions.

   d. Write in short 'double-reciprocal plot'.

   e. What are epimers? Explain by giving examples. Give the structures of epimers of D-glucose.

   f. What are disaccharides? Give the names of *two* reducing disaccharides. Mention their hydrolysis products.

Q 4. Solve any *four* of the following:

   a. Classify vitamins according to their solubilities with examples. Give biochemical role of vitamin B_6.

   b. Enumerate the role and deficiency symptoms of vitamin D?

   c. Give the different forms of vitamin A and vitamin K.

   d. Write short note on (any *one*):

      i. Transamination   ii. Oxidative deamination

   e. What are biochemical roles of calcium?

   f. Match the following:

I	II
i. Haemoglobin	1. Iodine
ii. The most abundant mineral in the body	2. Cobalt
iii. Enlargement of thyroid	3. Iron
iv. Relaxation of muscles	4. Calcium
v. Vitamin B_{12}	5. Sodium
	6. Zinc

Q 5. Solve any *two* of the following:

   a. Describe Krebs cycle. Discuss its significance.

   b. Give an account on metabolism of fats with reference to β-oxidation.

   c. Discuss in brief 'biosynthesis of urea'.

Q 6 Solve any *two* of the following:

   a. How acetone and blood is detected in urine?

   b. Name any *three* normal organic and *three* normal inorganic constituents of urine.

   c. Name the pathological conditions caused due to the presence of sugar, ketone, blood and protein in urine.

  d. Define:
    i. Iodine value
    ii. Acid value of lipids. Give their significance.
  e. Name and explain any *two* colour tests of proteins.
  f. Describe the role played by mitochondria.

Summer Examination 1999
D Pharm First Year
Biochemistry and Clinical Pathology

Q 1.
  a. Draw structures of fructose and galactose.
  b. Fill in the blanks:
    i. Vitamin _____ is required for blood coagulation.
    ii. Deficiency of haemoglobin in blood causes _____.
    iii. _____ and _____ are the coenzymes of riboflavin.
    iv. Deficiency of insulin results into a condition called _____.
    v. Deficiency of vitamin niacin causes _____.
    vi. Protein deficiency in infants below one year produces disease called _____.
  c. Answer in short:
    i. What is the use of iodine number?
    ii. What are ketone bodies?
    iii. What is an active site of enzyme?
    iv. What are α-amino acids?

Q 2.
  a. What is the biological value of proteins?
  b. Explain following test for proteins:
    i. Biuret test
    ii. Heat test
    iii. Test with trichloroacetic acid
  c. Write in short:
    Alkaptonuria and phenyl ketonuria

Q 3.
  a. What is the biological value of carbohydrates? How disaccharides are classified?
  b. Explain following tests:
    i. Benedict's test
    ii. Molisch's test
    iii. Fehling's test

Q 4. What are lipids? Give their classification with examples.

Q 5. Explain structure, biochemical role and deficiencies of vitamin 'D' or vitamin 'riboflavin'.

Q 6. Explain biochemical role of sodium and potassium and diseases caused by their deficiencies.

Q 7.

a. What are enzymes?

b. What is the effect of temperature, hydrogen ion concentration (pH) and substrate concentration on enzymatic reaction?

c. What is marker enzyme?

Q 8. Explain Krebs cycle and its bioenergetics.

Q 9. What are the abnormalities of red cell? Explain.

Q 10. Write notes on any *two*:

a. Urea cycle

b. Diabetes mellitus

c. Lipids in biological membrane

Winter Examination 1999
D Pharm First Year
Biochemistry and Clinical Pathology

Q 1. Attempt any *five* of the following:

a. Enumerate the essential and nonessential amino acids.

b. Mention the normal and abnormal constituents of urine.

c. Explain the role of vitamin D in brief.

d. Explain the disease scurvy. Give its causes.

e. Give the ring structure of α and BD glucose.

f. What do you understand by acid number of fats?

g. Give the α-helical structure of protein.

Q 2. Attempt any *two* of the following:

a. What are the carbohydrates? Give their classification.

b. Explain the formation of osazone of glucose and fructose and α and BD methyl glycoside.

c. What are the disaccharide? Describe the properties of lactose sugar.

d. Give the chemistry of Molisch's test and Benedict's solution test of carbohydrates.

Q 3. Attempt any *three* of the following:

a. What are the essential and nonessential α-amino acids? Give the structure of three amino acids of each class.

b. What is meant by isoelectric pH of α-amino acids and proteins? Give the isoelectric pH value of lysine and glycine.

c. State the biological importance and functions of protein.

d. Illustrate the medicinal significance of enzymes and their use for the manufacture of drugs.

Q 4. Attempt any *three* of the following:

a. What are the lipids? How are they classified? Give one example of each class.

b. How the lipids molecules are arrange in biological membrane? Explain the formation of lipid bilayer in membrane.

c. What are the phospholipids? Give their classification and general structure of phospholipids. Give one example of each class.

d. Write notes on:
   i. Phenyl ketonuria
   ii. Hyperglycaemia

Q 5. Attempt any *three* of the following:

a. Illustrate the biochemical role of vitamin C. Why it is essential? Difficiency of vitamin C causes which diseases.

b. State the important significance of folic acid or vitamin B_{12} for metabolism.

c. How the protein metabolism takes place in our body? Explain the process of metabolism.

d. Describe the electron transport and respirator chain.

e. Explain α-helical structure of protein.

Q 6. Attempt any *three* of the following:

a. Explain the Krebs cycle or citric acid cycle.

b. Define the terms catabolism, anabolism and glycolysis.

c. Explain the following disease and their causes:
   i. Diabetes mellitus
   ii. Pentosuria

d. Write short notes on (any *two*):
   i. Biosynthesis of urea
   ii. Bile salts
   iii. Prostaglandins

e. Explain the formation of peptides and polypeptides bonds in proteins.

Summer Examination 2000
D Pharm First Year
Biochemistry and Clinical Pathology

Q 1.

    a. Draw structures of glucose and galactose.

    b. Fill in the blanks:

        i. Vitamin _____ is essential for calcium absorption.

        ii. _____ and _____ are coenzymes of vitamin niacin.

        iii. _____ and _____ are mainly essential for water balance in body.

        iv. Deficiency of ascorbic acid causes _____.

        v. Bile salts and sex hormones are synthesized from _____.

        vi. Protein deficiency in children between the age of 1–4 years causes a disease _____.

    c. Answer in short:

        i. Complete and incomplete proteins.

        ii. Specificity of enzyme.

        iii. Hyperglycemia and hypoglycemia.

        iv. What is the use of iodine number?

Q 2.

    a. Define proteins.

    b. Explain following test of amino acids:

        i. Xanthoprotein test

        ii. Glyoxilic acid test

        iii. Ninhydrin test

    c. Explain the following protein deficiencies:

        i. Kwashiorkor   ii. Marasmus

Q 3. What are carbohydrates? Give their classification with examples.

Q 4.

    a. Define lipids. What are its functions?

    b. How simple lipids are classified?

    c. Write any one test for lipid.

Q 5. Explain the structure, biological role and deficiencies of vitamin 'A' or thiamine.

Q 6. Draw a well labelled diagram of Krebs cycle and describe. Explain its bioenergetics.

Q 7. Explain biochemical role of iron. What are the diseases causes by its deficiency? Explain.

Q 8.
a. What is the pharmacological importance of enzymes?
b. What is the effect of following factors on enzymatic reactions:
   i. Substrate concentration
   ii. Temperature
   iii. Hydrogen ion concentration

Q 9. What are the abnormal constituents in urine? Describe.

Q 10. Write note on (any *two*):
a. Ketone bodies
b. Marker enzymes
c. Inborn errors of protein metabolism.

Winter Examination 2000
D Pharm First Year
Biochemistry and Clinical Pathology

Q 1.
a. Draw a structure of glucose and fructose.
b. Fill in the blanks:
   i. Deficiency of vitamin A causes _____.
   ii. Deficiency of insulin leads to a condition called _____.
   iii. _____ is the coenzyme of vitamin thiamine.
   iv. _____ and _____ are the abnormal constituents in urine.
   v. Deficiency of vitamin _____ results into disease beriberi.
   vi. Protein deficiency in children between the ages of one to four years causes a disease called _____.
c. Answer in short:
   i. Specificity of enzyme.
   ii. Which bonds are responsible for primary structure of protein?
   iii. What are alpha-amino acids?
   iv. Any two examples of enzymes used in drug manufacturing.

Q 2.
a. What are proteins?
b. Explain following test of amino acid.
   i. Million's test
   ii. Sakaguchi test
   iii. Reanthoprotein test

   c. Explain following protein deficiencies:

      i. Marasmus   ii. Phenyl ketonuria

Q 3.

   a. What are carbohydrates? Explain. Classification of polysaccharide only.

   b. Osazone test.

Q 4.

   a. Define saponification value and iodine number.

   b. Describe classification of compound lipids only.

Q 5. Explain structure, biochemical role and deficiencies of vitamin 'A' or nicotinic acid.

Q 6. Explain biochemical role of calcium and diseases caused by calcium deficiency.

Q 7. What are enzymes? How they are classified?

Q 8. Describe glycolytic pathway along with its bioenergetics.

Q 9. What are the abnormalities of red cells? Explain.

Q 10. Write notes on (any *two*):

   a. Marker enzymes

   b. Diabetes mellitus

   c. Ketone bodies

Summer Examination 2001
D Pharm First Year
Biochemistry and Clinical Pathology

Q 1. Solve any *five* of the following:

   a. Define the following terms with significance.

      i. Iodine number   ii. Saponification number

   b. What are reducing sugars? Give the structures of D-glucose and D-fructose.

   c. Describe the following (any *two*):

      i. Cori cycle   iii. Diabetes mellitus

      ii. Maple syrup disease

   d. Give the physiological functions, deficiency symptoms and the structure of ascorbic acid or niacin.

   e. What are essential amino acids? Give example and draw the structure of phenyl alanine.

   f. Discuss the oxidation reactions of D-glucose.

   g. What are isoenzymes and marker enzymes?

Q 2. Solve any *three* of the following:

   a. Explain: "Role of lipids in biological membranes".

   b. Define— 'enzyme inhibition'. Mention their different types. Explain—allosteric inhibition.

   c. Define and classify vitamins. Name the deficiency disease of thiamine and folic acid.

   d. What are simple proteins? Mention the biological functions of proteins.

   e. What are the functions and deficiency symptoms of other following (any *two*):

      i. Iron   iii. Potassium

      ii. Sodium

Q 3. Solve any *three* of the following:

   a. Give the different forms of vitamin A. How are they derived? Mention the functions and deficiency of diseases of vitamin A.

   b. What are oligosaccharides? Name three important disaccharides with their hydrolysis products.

   c. Define and classify amino acids.

   d. Name the factors that affect the velocity of the enzyme catalysed reactions. Describe the effect of the pH on enzyme reaction.

   e. Explain— 'electron transport chain'.

Q 4. Solve any *three* of the following:

   a. Define phospholipids, and classify them with examples.

   b. What are polysaccharides? Give the different types and functions.

   c. Discuss the diagnostic applications of enzymes.

   d. What are trace-elements? Give their examples. Give the physiological functions and deficiency diseases of iodine.

   e. Explain the following reactions of proteins.

      i. Biuret test   ii. Xanthoproteic test

Q 5. Solve any *three* of the following:

   a. Describe the two main compartments in which water in human body is distributed. Mention the physiological functions of water in the human body.

   b. What are the main abnormal constituents of urine? Define the terms:

      i. Proteinuria   ii. Glycosuria

   c. Define anaemia. What is microcytic anaemia? How it is treated?

   d. Explain the following (any *two*):

      i. Nieman-Pick's disease

      ii. Kwashiorkor

      iii. Mechanism of enzyme action

   e. Define the following terms:

      i. Rickets   iii. Polycythemia

      ii. Egg white injury   iv. Leucocytosis

Q 6. Solve any *two* of the following:

   a. Define glycolysis. Explain reactions involved in it.

   b. What do you understand by beta-oxidation? Give the reactions of beta-oxidation of fatty acid.

   c. Explain the following reactions of protein metabolism.

      i. Transamination

      ii. Deamination

      iii. Decarboxylation

Winter Examination 2001
D Pharm First Year
Biochemistry and Clinical Pathology

Q 1. Solve any *five* of the following:

   a. Explain acid-base behaviour of amino acids.

   b. Define biochemistry and give its importance.

   c. What is active site of enzyme?

   d. Define with example:

      i. Reducing sugar

      ii. Oligosaccharide

   e. Name the normal constituent of urine.

   f. Explain proteins briefly.

   g. Give the biological function of lipids.

Q 2. Solve any *four* of the following:

   a. What are disaccharides? Give its example and mention their hydrolysis product.

   b. Write short note on competitive inhibition.

   c. Name the vitamins belonging to B-complex group.

   d. Explain essential fatty acids. Give its example.

   e. What are erythrocytes? Explain.

   f. Explain primary structure of proteins.

Q 3. Solve any *four* of the following:

    a. Name the diseases which occur due to disorder of lipid metabolism. Explain any one.

    b. Discuss in brief concept of enzyme action.

    c. Classify proteins with examples.

    d. Give the properties, structure and use of sucrose.

    e. Explain the biochemical role of iron.

    f. Write a short note on triglycerides.

Q 4. Solve any *four* of the following:

    a. Give the oxidation product of glucose with difference oxidising agent.

    b. Name the deficiency disease of following vitamins.

        i. Calciferol   v. Niacin

        ii. Retinol   vi. Phylloquinone

       iii. Ascorbic acid   vii. Cynocobalamin

       iv. Thiamine

    c. Define:

        i. Acid value   iii. Polensky number

       ii. Richert-Missel number

    d. Explain biuret test and ninhydrin test of proteins.

    e. Match the following:

        i. Enlargement of thyroid   1. Calcium

       ii. Vitamin B_{12} 2. Iodine

      iii. The most abundant mineral   3. Cobalt

           in body   4. Phosphorus

    f. Give the structure of (any *three*):

        i. Linoleic acid   iii. Cholesterol

       ii. Stearic acid   iv. Arachidonic acid

Q 5. Solve any *four* of the following:

    a. How acetone and blood is detected in urine?

    b. Describe the role played by mitochondria.

    c. Explain biological function of proteins.

    d. What are fats and oils? Discuss their physical and chemical properties.

    e. Explain briefly enzyme specificity.

    f. What are amino acids? Give the structure of aromatic amino acids.

Q 6. Solve any *four* of the following:

    a. Describe the Krebs cycle.

    b. Explain the biosynthesis of urea.

    c. Discuss in brief the reaction involved in glycolysis.

   d. Explain the role of vitamin A in vision.

   e. Explain B-oxidation of fatty acids.

   f. What is phenyl ketonuria and alkaptonuria?

Summer Examination 2002
D Pharm First Year
Biochemistry and Clinical Pathology

Q 1. Solve any *five* of the following:

   a. Define and classify carbohydrates on chemical basis.

   b. Give the different factors affecting on enzyme catalysed reaction. Explain any *two* of them.

   c. Explain the biological function of vitamin D.

   d. What are minerals and give their major function in life processes?

   e. What are platelets? Explain. ·

   f. Give the structure and *two* colour test of cholesterol.

   g. Explain qualitative test of proteins.

Q 2. Solve any *four* of the following:

   a. What are essential amino acids. Give its examples.

   b. Give two identification test of reducing sugar.

   c. Explain water balance of body.

   d. What are enzymes give their major classification?

   e. Draw the structure of:

      i. D-glucose   iii. Lactose

      ii. Sucrose

   f. Discuss the peptide bond of protein.

Q 3. Solve any *four* of the following:

   a. Write a short note on role of calcium in life processes.

   b. Explain the principle of following test:

      i. Molisch's test   ii. Fehling's test

   c. Describe the role played by cell nucleus.

   d. Define the terms:

      i. Saponification value   iii. Isoenzyme

      ii. Metalloenzyme

   e. Explain following terms:

      i. Prosthetic group   iii. Isoenzyme

      ii. Metalloenzyme

   f. Explain following biochemical processes:

      i. Transamination   ii. Deamination

Q 4. Solve any *four* of the following:

a. What are lipids? Classify with examples.

b. Define anaemia. Explain megaloblastic anaemia.

c. What is action of dilute alkali or glucose?

d. Define and classify vitamins. Name the vitamins belonging to B-complex group.

e. What are leucocytes? Give different types of leucocytes.

f. Define the terms:

i. Catabolism   iii. Abnormal metabolism

ii. Metabolism

Q 5. Solve any *two* of the following:

a. Describe in brief the reaction involved in beta-oxidation.

b. Describe the TCA cycle.

c. Describe in brief the reaction involved in glycolysis.

Q 6. Solve any *four* of the following:

a. Define coenzyme. Name the coenzyme of:

i. Niacin   ii. Folic acid

b. Name the abnormal constituent present in urine and give their significance disease.

c. Give the pharmaceutical importance of enzyme.

d. Name the protein deficiency disease. Explain (any *one*).

e. How protein and blood is detected in urine?

f. i. Cobalt containing vitamin is _____.

ii. Except _____ all the amino acids are optically active.

iii. Goiter is disease cause due to deficiency of _____ mineral.

Winter Examination 2002
D Pharm First Year
Biochemistry and Clinical Pathology

Q 1. Solve any *five* of the following:

a. Define the following terms:

i. Glycogenesis   iii. Gluconeogenesis

ii. Glycogenolysis   iv. Glycolysis

b. What are essential fatty acids? Give their examples.

c. Explain—mutarotation. Give the structure of α and β-D-glucose.

d. Describe in brief:

i. Phenylketonuria   ii. Alkaptonuria

   e. What are lipids? Give their biological importance.

   f. Define and classify vitamins with examples. Draw the structure of pyridoxine.

   g. What are enzymes? Mention their six major classes.

Q 2. Solve any *three* of the following:

   a. Discuss primary and secondary structure of proteins.

   b. Explain the role of vitamin A in vision. Give deficiency diseases of vitamin A.

   c. What are coenzymes? Illustrate with examples.

   d. Give the biological role of (any *two*):

      i. Calcium   iii. Phosphorus

      ii. Iron

   e. Explain the following tests of carbohydrates:

      i. Molisch's test   ii. Benedict's test

Q 3. Solve any *three* of the following:

   a. Define carbohydrates and classify them with examples.

   b. Discuss the role of lipids in biological membranes.

   c. Explain any *two* of the following:

      i. Denaturation of proteins   iii. Conjugated proteins

      ii. Biuret test of proteins

   d. Mention different factors affecting enzyme catalysed reactions. What is the effect of temperature on enzyme action?

   e. Explain "lock and key" model of enzyme action. Give Michalis-Menten equation and define 'K_m'.

Q 4. Solve any *three* of the following:

   a. Enumerate the role and deficiency symptoms of:

      i. Vitamin C   ii. Vitamin D

   b. Explain water balance of the body.

   c. Define anaemia. What is megaloblastic anaemia? How it is treated?

   d. Define abnormal urine. Enlist the abnormal constituents of urine with their corresponding diseases.

   e. What are steroids? Give their examples. Give the examples of any *two* saturated and unsaturated fatty acids.

Q 5. Solve any *three* of the following:

   a. Explain (any *two*).

      i. Acid-base behaviour of amino acids

      ii. Biological functions of proteins

      iii. Dietary deficiency of proteins

   b. Define the following with examples.

      i. Anomers   ii. Epimers

c. Give the therapeutic and pharmaceutical importance of enzymes.

d. What are minerals? Classify them giving examples.

e. What are α-amino acids? Give the examples of any *two* sulphur containing amino acids. What is isoelectric pH of an amino acid?

Q 6. Solve any *two* of the following:

a. Discuss in brief reactions involved in glycolysis.

b. Explain beta-oxidation of fatty acids.

c. Describe the reactions of urea cycle.

Summer Examination 2003
D Pharm First Year
Biochemistry and Clinical Pathology

Q 1. Solve any *ten* of the following:

a. What are conjugated proteins? Give its examples.

b. Define with suitable example:

    i. Induced enzyme   ii. Constitutive enzyme

c. Describe role of water in life processes.

d. Name the vitamins belonging to B-complex group.

e. Describe the role played by cell nucleus.

f. Enumerate the abnormal constituents of urine. Give their significance in diseases.

g. Define lipids. Give their biological importance.

h. Explain the identification test of proteins.

i. What are carbohydrates. Give its classification on basis of solubility with example.

j. Define coenzyme.

    Give the coenzyme of:

    i. Folic acid   ii. Thiamine

k. What are minerals? Give their classification with example.

l. Explain mutarotation.

Q 2. Solve any *four* of the following:

a. Write the structure of cholesterol. Give its colour test.

b. Discuss in brief, concept of enzyme action.

c. What are monosaccharides? Explain and give its example.

d. Name the protein deficiency diseases. Explain any *one*.

e. What are leucocytes? Give the different types of leucocytes.

f. Explain water balance of normal individual.

Q 3. Solve any *four* of the following:

   a. Give the clinical applications of enzymes.

   b. Define:

      i. Acetyl value

      ii. Saponification value

   c. Give the principle of Molisch's test.

   d. Define:

      i. Catabolism

      ii. Anabolism

      iii. Abnormal metabolism

   e. What is blood and give the function of blood.

   f. Explain the biological importance of vitamin D.

Q 4. Solve any *four* of the following:

   a. What is sucrose. Give its structure and properties.

   b. What are essential amino acids? Give examples.

   c. Discuss the qualitative tests of lipids.

   d. Explain the biological importance of vitamin C.

   e. Explain the terms:

      i. Rickets

      ii. Osteoporosis

   f. Give the reactions of following reagents with amino acids.

      i. FDNB

      ii. Dansyl chloride

      iii. Dansyl chlorides—this reagent is used to determine the N-terminal amino acid residue of polypeptides. The amino group of free amino acid also reacts with dansyl chloride.

Q 5. Solve any *four* of the following:

   a. Give the difference between competitive and noncompetitive inhibition.

   b. Discuss the role of calcium in life processes.

   c. How sugar and bile salt is detected in urine?

   d. Discuss the formation of osazone of glucose.

   e. Describe the role played by mitochondria.

   f. Discuss the denaturation of proteins briefly.

Q 6. Solve any *three* of the following:

   a. Outline the steps involved in urea cycle.

   b. Describe the electron transport and respiratory chain.

   c. Describe in brief ketosis.

   d. Explain role of vitamin A in vision.

   e. Discuss in brief β-oxidation of fatty acid.

Winter Examination 2003
D Pharm First Year
Biochemistry and Clinical Pathology

Q 1. Solve any *five* of the following.

    a. Explain secondary structure of proteins.

    b. Discuss the major intracellular organs and their function.

    c. Give the structure of (any *four*):

i. D-glucose	iv. Sucrose
ii. Lactose	v. Fructose
iii. Maltose	

    d. Define following (any *four*):

i. Acid value	iv. Reichert-Meissel number
ii. Saponification value	v. Acetyl number
iii. Iodine number	

    e. What is:

i. Glycogenesis	iii. Gluconeogenesis
ii. Glycogenolysis	iv. Glycolysis

    f. Name the respective vitamin responsible for nutritional deficiency cause:

i. Pellagra	v. Night-blindness
ii. Blood clotting disorder	vi. Pernicious anaemia
iii. Beriberi	vii. Scurvy
iv. Rickets	viii. Nutritional anaemia

    g. Enlist the normal and abnormal constituents of urine.

Q 2. Solve any *two* of the following:

    a. Name the factors which affect rate of enzyme catalysed reaction. Explain any three factors.

    b. What are carbohydrates? Classify them with suitable examples.

    c. Explain the structure. Biochemical role and deficiency diseases of vitamin A or niacin.

Q 3. Solve any *two* of the following:

    a. What are fats and oils? Discuss their physical and chemical properties briefly.

    b. Define proteins and give their biological functions. Classify them on chemical composition with example.

    c. Describe in brief the reactions involved in glycolysis.

Q 4. Solve any *two* of the following:

a. Name the vitamins belonging to B-complex group. Give their respective coenzyme and function.

b. Discuss the properties of water in body and explain water balance of normal individual.

c. Describe in brief the reactions involved in beta-oxidation.

Q 5. Solve any *two* of the following:

a. Discuss the following reactions of monosaccharides.
   i. Osazone formation
   ii. Oxidation

b. What are essential fatty acids? Give examples with structure.

c. What are abnormalities of red blood cell? Explain.

Q 6. Solve any *two* of the following:

a. Define and classify amino acids with examples. Write structure of one of the aromatic amino acids.

b. Give one function and one deficiency symptom of:
   i. Iron   iii. Iodine
   ii. Potassium

c. Define with example (any *four*):
   i. Endoenzyme   iv. Constitutive enzyme
   ii. Exoenzyme   v. Induced enzyme
   iii. Isoenzyme   vi. Activators

Summer Examination 2004
D Pharm First Year
Biochemistry and Clinical Pathology

Q 1. Solve any *five* of the following:

a. What do you mean by metabolism, anabolism, catabolism and glycosuria?

b. Explain 'denaturation of proteins.
   Define:
   i. Proteinuria   ii. Biochemistry

c. Give brief idea about AIDS.

d. Explain the terms with their significances.
   i. Acid value   ii. Acetyl value

e. Desceibe in brief, megaloblastic and pernicious anaemia.

f. Explain:
   i. Osazone formation   ii. Glycosidic linkage
g. What are vitamins? Classify them with examples.
   Define 'beriberi'

Q 2. Solve any *three* of the following:

a. Explain the following:
   i. Molisch's test   ii. Benedict's test
b. What are lipids? Give brief classification with examples.
c. Discuss acid-base behaviours of amino acids.
d. What are simple and conjugated proteins? Mention biological functions of proteins.
e. Explain in brief role of vitamin D in body. Give its deficiency diseases.

Q 3. Solve any *three* of the following:

a. Explain in brief water balance in human body.
b. What are reducing and nonreducing carbohydrates? How do they differ from each other?
c. Explain 'kwashiorkor' and 'marasmus' diseases.
d. Give physiological role of iodine and zinc.
e. What are essential fatty acids? Explain with examples.

Q 4. Solve any *three* of the following:

a. Discuss in brief secondary structure of proteins.
b. Classify carbohydrates with examples.
c. Name different factors affecting rate of enzyme action. Explain the effect of enzyme concentration and temperature.
d. Define the terms:
   i. Holoenzymes   iii. Coenzymes
   ii. Apoenzymes   iv. Zymogens
e. What are trace elements? Give physiological functions and deficiency diseases of iron.

Q 5. Solve any *three* of the following:

a. Explain:
   i. Phenylketonuria   ii. Maple-syrup disease
b. What are ketone-bodies? Explain ketosis.
c. Explain 'deamination' and 'decarboxylation' process in protein metabolism.
d. Enlist the abnormal constituents of urine. Name the conditions in which they appear.
e. What are coenzymes? Explain with examples.

Q 6. Solve any *two* of the following:
- a. Explain in brief reactions involved in 'TCA' cycle.
- b. Describe formation of urea in protein metabolism.
- c. Give an account of metabolism of fats with reference to β-oxidation.

Winter Examination 2004
D Pharm First Year
Biochemistry and Clinical Pathology

Q 1. Attempt any *five* of the following:
- a. Define the following terms with significance:
    - i. Acid value
    - ii. Iodine number
- b. What are carbohydrates? Give structures of:
    - i. D-glucose
    - ii. D-fructose
- c. Describe the following:
    - i. Glycogen storage diseases
    - ii. Diabetes mellitus
- d. Define the term 'essential amino acids'. Mention any *four* of them.
- e. What are 'essential fatty acids'? Give their examples.
- f. Define with suitable examples:
    - i. Induced enzymes
    - ii. Constitutional enzymes
- g. Describe the role of water in life processes.

Q 2. Attempt any *three* of the following:
- a. Explain the following tests:
    - i. Rothera's test
    - ii. Liberman-Burchard reaction
- b. Name protein deficiency diseases. Explain any *one* of them.
- c. What are lymphocytes. Give their role in health and disease.
- d. Explain water balance of normal individual.
- e. Discuss osazone formation test for glucose.

Q 3. Attempt any *three* of the following:
- a. Explain the following terms:
    - i. Rickets
    - ii. Osteoporosis
- b. Give reactions of following reagents with amino acids:
    - i. FDNB
    - ii. Dansyl chloride
- c. Define the following with examples.
    - i. Anomers
    - ii. Epimers
- d. How will you detect the following from the given sample of urine?
    - i. Sugar
    - ii. Blood
- e. Define lipids. Give their biological importance.

Q 4. Attempt any *three* of the following:

    a. Define the term 'coenzymes'. Name the coenzymes obtained from:

        i. Folic acid   iii. Pentothenic acid

        ii. Thiamine

    b. Explain biochemical role and deficiency symptoms of:

        i. Iodine   ii. Zinc

    c. Describe the role played by "mitochondria".

    d. Enlist various factors affecting rate of enzymic reaction. State the effect of:

        i. pH

        ii. Temperature on enzyme catalysed reaction

    e. Name the vitamin; deficiency of which leads to:

        i. Egg white injury   iii. Pernicious anaemia

        ii. Microcytic anaemia   iv. Beriberi

Q 5. Attempt any *three* of the following:

    a. State abnormal constituents of urine. Name the conditions in which they appear.

    b. Explain:

        i. Alkaptonuria   ii. Phenylketonuria

    c. Describe the role of lipids in biological membrane.

    d. Define the following terms:

        i. Glycogenesis   iii. Glucogenolysis

        ii. Glycogenolysis   iv. Purpura

    e. Explain mutarotation with suitable example.

Q 6. Attempt any *two* of the following:

    a. Discuss in brief reactions involved in glycolysis. Give its bioenergetics.

    b. Explain beta-oxidation of fatty acids.

    c. Describe the reactions of urea cycle.

Summer Examination 2005
D Pharm First Year
Biochemistry and Clinical Pathology

Q 1. Solve any *five* of the following.

    a. Explain the following terms:

        i. Kwashiorkor   iii. Jaundice

        ii. Leucocytosis   iv. Anuria

b. Give structures of the following:
    i. D-glucose   iii. D-galactose
    ii. D-fructose   iv. D-mannose

c. Give a neat labelled diagram of a typical animal cell. Give the functions of:
    i. Cell membrane   ii. Mitochondria

d. What are proteins? Explain α-helix structure of proteins.

e. Define simple lipids. Classify simple lipids with examples. Differentiate between oils and fats.

f. Give structure and biological functions of folic acid.

g. Define:
    i. Multienzyme complex   iii. Inductive enzymes
    ii. Isoenzyme   iv. Zymogens

Q 2. Solve any *three* of the following:

a. Enlist the factors affecting the rate of enzyme catalysed reaction. Describe in detail the effect of substrate.

b. Explain the biological functions and the factors affecting the rate of absorption of calcium in the body.

c. Explain the following reactions of protein metabolism:
    i. Deamination   ii. Transamination

d. Define abnormal urine. Give any six abnormal constituents of urine with the ailment associated with them.

e. Explain the role of vitamin A in vision.

Q 3. Solve any *three* of the following:

a. Define anaemia. Explain sickle-cell anaemia.

b. What is beta-oxidation of fatty acids? Give reactions of beta-oxidation of fatty acids.

c. Explain the following:
    i. Abnormal metabolism   iii. Catabolism
    ii. Metabolism   iv. Anabolism

d. Explain acid-base behaviour of proteins.

e. Give the therapeutic and pharmaceutical importance of enzymes.

Q 4. Solve any *three* of the following:

a. Explain in detail the urea cycle in protein metabolism.

b. Explain 'lock and key' model and 'induced fil' model of mechanism of enzyme action.

c. Describe the following:
    i. Phenylketonuria   ii. Maple syrup disease

d. Classify minerals. Give physiological functions of minerals.

    e. Explain the osazone formation of carbohydrates with significance of the reaction.

Q 5. Solve any *three* of the following:

    a. Explain any *two* of the following:
        i. Mucosal block theory of iron absorption
        ii. Rickets
        iii. Hypokalaemia

    b. Write a note on polysaccharides.

    c. Define and classify vitamins. Name the vitamins belonging to B-complex groups.

    d. Explain the biological functions of lipids.

    e. Give chemical names of vitamins K_1 and K_2. Give biological functions of vitamin K.

Q 6. Solve any *three* of the following:

    a. What are lipids? Classify compound lipids with examples.

    b. Give the steps involved in the Krebs cycle with the enzymes involved at each step.

    c. Define amino acids. Give structure of:
        i. Aromatic amino acid
        ii. Optically inactive amino acid
        iii. Acidic amino acid

    d. Explain glycogenesis and glycogenolysis.

    e. Give the following test:
        i. Ninhydrin test   iii. Salkowaski's test
        ii. Molisch's test   iv. Xanthoprotein test

Winter Examination 2005
D Pharm First Year
Biochemistry and Clinical Pathology

Q 1. Solve any *five* of the following.

    a. Define:
        i. Biochemistry and biomolecules
        ii. Anabolism and catabolism

    b. What are normal and abnormal constitutents of urine? Give examples of each.

    c.   i. What is anaemia? Enlist its types.
        ii. Define leucocytes and give types of leucocytes.

    d. Explain 'mutarotation'.

   e. Give the structure and role of miochondria in cell.

   f. Define the following giving their significance:

      i. Iodine value

      ii. Saponification value

   g. Give the structures of the following:

      i. D-glucose   iii. Niacin

      ii. D-fructose   iv. Pyridoxine

Q 2. Solve any *three* of the following:

   a. Define carbohydrates. Classify them with examples.

   b. Explain the role of lipids in biological membrane.

   c. Describe any *two* colour tests for proteins.

   d. Mention different factors affecting rate of enzyme catalysed reactions. Explain the effect of temperature and pH.

   e. Give the examples of fat soluble vitamins. Explain role of vitamin 'A' in vision.

Q 3. Solve any *three* of the following:

   a. Give the compartments in which water in human is distributed. Write the importance of water in biological system.

   b. Differentiate between:

      i. Reducing and nonreducing sugars

      ii. Epimers and anomers

   c. What are α-amino acids? Classify them with examples.

   d. Give the physiological role of sodium and zinc.

   e. Explain the following:

      i. Essential fatty acids

      ii. Rancidification of fats and oils

Q 4. Solve any *three* of the following:

   a. What are enzymes? Explain competitive inhibition.

   b. Define the terms:

      i. Coenzymes

      ii. Isoenzymes

      iii. Xerophthalmia

      iv. Scurvy

   c. What are minerals? Give physiological functions of minerals.

   d. Explain:

      i. Essential amino acids

      ii. Primary structure of protein

   e. What are disaccharides? Give three examples with their hydrolysis products.

Q 5. Solve any *three* of the following:

    a. Define the terms:

        i. Glycogenesis   iii. Ketosis

        ii. Gluconeogenesis   iv. Hyperglycaemia

    b. Explain 'transamination' process in protein metabolism.

    c. Name any *two* inborn errors of protein metabolism. Explain 'alkaptonuria'.

    d. How sugars and proteins are detected in urine? Name the conditions in which they appear.

    e. Explain:

        i. Arteriosclerosis   ii. Niemann-Pick disease

Q 6. Solve any *two* of the following:

    a. Explain the reactions involved in 'glycolysis'.

    b. Describe β-oxidation of fatty acids.

    c. Explain in brief the reactions of 'urea cycle'.

Summer Examination 2006
D Pharm First Year
Biochemistry and Clinical Pathology

Q 1. Solve any *five* of the following.

    a. Draw a neat labelled diagram of a typical animal cell and describe functions of mitochondria.

    b. Give structures of the following:

        i. α-D-glucose   iii. Maltose

        ii. β-D-fructose   iv. Sucrose

    c. Explain secondary structure of proteins.

    d. Discuss biological role of lipids.

    e. What are minerals? Classify them with example (define each class and subclass).

    f. Define the following:

        i. Isoenzymes   iii. Adoptive enzymes

        ii. Multienzymes   iv. Constitutive enzymes

    g. What is glycolysis? Give steps involved in the process of glycolysis.

Q 2. Solve any *three* of the following:

    a. Explain oxazone formation in carbohydrates. Give its significance.

    b. Explain:

        i. Sucrose is nonreducing sugar

        ii. Maltose is reducing sugar

   c. Give following reactions of amino acids with their significance.

      i. Ninhydrin reaction   ii. Edman's reaction

   d. Define the following for lipids.

      i. Acid value   iii. Polensky value

      ii. Sap value   iv. Iodine value

   e. What is anaemia? Describe pernicious anaemia and sickle-cell anaemia.

Q 3. Solve any *three* of the following:

   a. Give classification of enzymes, based on main types of biochemical reactions.

   b. What is pathological urine? Give significance of abnormal constituents of urine.

   c. Discuss the following reactions with their importance.

      i. Oxidative deamination   ii. Transamination

   d. Explain role of lipids in biological membrane with reference to Danielli and Davison's model and SJ Singer's model.

   e. Give structure and colour reactions of cholesterol.

Q 4. Solve any *three* of the following:

   a. Give structure, biological active form and biological functions of vitamin B_1.

   b. Explain factors affecting absorptions of 'Fe' and also give biological functions of 'Fe'.

   c. Give the factors affecting rate of enzyme catalysed reaction. Discuss in detail effect of substrate with equations and curves.

   d. Define and explain the process of ketogenesis and ketogenolysis.

   e. Define the following terms:

      i. Lymphocytosis   iii. Anuria

      ii. Thrombocytopaenia   iv. Glycosuria

Q 5. Solve any *three* of the following:

   a. Compare between the following:

      i. Competitive inhibition and noncompetitive inhibition.

      ii. Lock and key mechanism and induced fit mechanism of enzyme action.

   b. Write in short about:

      i. Rhodopsin cycle   ii. Pellagra

   c. What are phospholipids? Give structure and biological function of lecithins.

   d. What are proteins? Classify proteins with example (give definition of each class and subclass).

e. Explain the following rections:
   i. Molisch's test   iii. Barfoed's test
   ii. Xanthoprotein test   iv. Biuret test

Q 6. Solve any *two* of the following:
   a. Explain in brief the reactions of Krebs cycle.
   b. Explain in brief the reactions involved in extramitochondrial synthesis of fatty acids.
   c. Explain in brief the reactions of urea cycle.

Winter Examination 2006
D Pharm First Year
Biochemistry and Clinical Pathology

Q 1. Solve any *five* of the following.
   a. Define the following terms with examples.
      i. Reducing sugars   iii. Phospholipids
      ii. Essential amino acids   iv. Isoenzymes
   b. Give structures of following:
      i. Lactose   iii. Glycine
      ii. Amylose   iv. Tripalmitin
   c. Explain protein deficiency diseases.
   d. Discuss the effect of following on the rate of enzymes catalysed reactions.
      i. Substrate concentration   ii. Temperature
   e. What are vitamins? Classify them with examples.
   f. Give the meaning of following terms:
      i. Hyperglycaemia   iii. Polydypsia
      ii. Glycosuria   iv. Polyuria
   g. Define the following:
      i. Glycolysis   iii. Glycogenolysis
      ii. Glycogenesis   iv. Gluconeogenesis

Q 2. Solve any *three* of the following:
   a. Give the following reactions of glucose.
      i. Reduction   iii. Alkaline interconversion
      ii. Dehydration   iv. Osazone formation
   b. What are carbohydrates? Classify carbohydrates with examples.
   c. What are physiological and pathological constructions of urine? Discuss in brief diagnostic importance of pathological constituents of urine.

d. Define the term 'enzymes". How they are classified? Give examples of each class.

e. What are fixed oils and fats? Explain saponification and rancidification of oils.

Q 3. Solve any *three* of the following:

a. Explain:
    i. Alkaptonuria   ii. Phenylketonuria

b. Discuss competitive and noncompetitive inhibition and enzymes.

c. Give the structure, biochemical role and deficiency diseases of nicotinic acid.

d. Define the term "anemia". Explain megaloblastic anemia and sickle cell anemia.

e. Explain biological functions of calcium and iron in the body.

Q 4. Solve any *three* of the following:

a. Explain "mutarotation" of D-glucose. Give the structure of anomers of glucose.

b. Define the following terms:
    i. Acid value   iii. Reichert-Miessl number
    ii. Saponification value   iv. Iodine number

c. Discuss the diagnostic and therapeutic applications of enzymes.

d. Explain the following reactions:
    i. Benedict's test
    ii. Biuret test
    iii. Ninhydrin test
    iv. Libermann-Burchard reaction

e. Give the functions of following:
    i. Vitamin A   ii. Vitamin E

Q 5. Solve any *three* of the following:

a. What are coenzymes? Explain the biochemical role of coenzymes of riboflavin and pyridoxine.

b. Write a short account of:
    i. Beriberi   ii. Pellagra

c. What are lipids? Classify lipids with examples. Give one structure each of saturated and unsaturated fatty acids.

d. Discuss the mechanism of action enzymes.

e. Explain urea cycle.

Q 6. Solve any *two* of the followings:

a. Give the reactions involved in TCA cycle. Discuss its energetics.

b. Explain "electron transport chain".

c. Discuss beta-oxidation of fatty acids. Give its energetics by taking example of palmitic acid.

Summer Examination 2007
D Pharm First Year
Biochemistry and Clinical Pathology

Q 1. Solve any *five* of the following.

a. What do you mean by metabolism, anabolism, catabolism and glycosuria?

b. Define carbohydrates. Classify them with suitable examples. Give *four* properties of reducing sugars.

c. Give the structure of:
   - i. Maltose
   - iii. Sucrose
   - ii. Lactose

d. Draw a neat labeled diagram of a typical animal cell. Give the functions of mitochondria.

e. What are normal and abnormal constituents of urine? Mention abnormal constituents of urine and their significance in disease.

f. i. What is anaemia? Enlist its types.
   ii. Define leucocytes and give types of leucocytes.

g. Write the reaction involved in the formation of glucosazone.

Q 2. Solve any *three* of the following:

a. Explain acid-base behaviour of amino acids.

b. Enlist the factors affecting the rate of enzyme catalysed reaction. Describe in detail the effect of pH.

c. Explain in brief water balance in human body.

d. What are essential and nonessential amino acids? Discuss with examples.

e. Explain the role of lipids in biological membrane.

Q 3. Solve any *three* of the following:

a. Define dissacharides. Give the sources and uses of maltose and lactose.

b. Explain 'lock and key' model and 'induced fit' model of mechanism of enzyme action.

c. Write principles involved in colour tests for proteins.

d. What are trace elements? Give physiological functions and deficiency diseases of iron.

e. Explain in brief secondary structure of proteins.

Q 4. Solve any *three* of the following:
- a. Write inversion test for sucrose with its hydrolysis products.
- b. Define the terms:
    - i. Coenzymes
    - ii. Isoenzymes
    - iii. Acetyl number
    - iv. Reichert-Miessl number
- c. Explain the role of vitamin A in vision.
- d. Describe the following:
    - i. Phenylketonuria   ii. Maple syrup diseases
- e. Explain Rhodopsin cycle for vision.

Q 5. Solve any *three* of the following:
- a. What are ketone bodies? Explain ketosis.
- b. What are essential fatty acids? Explain with examples.
- c. Give the structure and colour reactions for cholesterol.
- d. Give the following test (only principles):
    - i. Molish test   ii. Iodine test
- e. What is mean by:
    - i. Glycogenesis   iii. Gluconeogenesis
    - ii. Glycolysis   iv. Glycogenolysis

Q 6. Solve any *two* of the following:
- a. Explain in brief reactions involved in 'TCA' cycle.
- b. Give an account of metabolism of fats with reference to β-oxidations.
- c. Define and classify amino acids with examples. Write structure of one aromatic amino acids.

Winter Examination 2007
D Pharm First Year
Biochemistry and Clinical Pathology

Q 1. Solve any *five* of the following.
- a. What do you mean by hyperglycaemia, Glycosuria, Proteinuria and haematuria?
- b. Explain the terms with their significance:
    - i. Saponification value   ii. Iodine value
- c. Describe in brief alkaptonuria and phenylketonuria.
- d. Define and classify carbohydrates with examples.
- e. Discuss the diagnostic and clinical applications of enzymes.

 f. Give the structures of:

   i. Maltose   iii. Sucrose

   ii. Lactose   iv. Fructose

 g. Explain acid-base behaviour of amino acids.

Q 2. Solve any *three* of the following:

 a. What are fatty acids? How they are classified? Define essential fatty acids.

 b. Explain the diseases caused by dietary deficiency of proteins.

 c. What is mutarotation? Give the structures of anomers of glucose.

 d. Explain the followings:

   i. Osazone test   ii. Benedict test

 e. What are proteins? Mention biological functions of proteins. Define essential amino acids.

Q 3. Solve any *three* of the following:

 a. Define and classify enzymes with examples.

 b. Explain role of vitamin A in the body. Give its deficiency diseases.

 c. Discuss secondary structures of proteins.

 d. Explain:

   i. Diabetes mellitus   ii. Artherosclerosis

 e. Explain 'transamination' and 'deamination' process in protein metabolism.

Q 4. Solve any *three* of the following:

 a. Explain the effect of pH and temperature on the rate of enzyme catalysed reactions.

 b. Define the terms:

   i. Denaturation   iii. Vitamins

   ii. Acid number   iv. Isoenzymes

 c. Discuss in brief any *two* of the following:

   i. Beriberi   iii. Scurvy

   ii. Egg white injury

 d. Describe megaloblastic and sickle cell anaemia.

 e. Write the mechanism of 'Fe' absorption and explain factors affecting absorption.

Q 5. Solve any *three* of the following:

 a. What is enzyme inhibition? Explain competitive inhibition with examples.

 b. Give the structure, biochemical role and deficiency diseases of nicotinic acid.

 c. Discuss pathology of lymphocytes and thrombocytes.

d. What are electrolytes? Explain their functions in the body.

e. Give an account of beta-oxidation of fatty acids.

Q 6. Solve any *two* of the following:

a. Explain in brief glycolysis.

b. Discuss 'TCA' cycle along with its energetics.

c. Describe "electron transport chain".

Summer Examination 2008
D Pharm First Year
Biochemistry and Clinical Pathology

Q 1. Solve any *five* of the following.

a. Define:

i.	Enzymes	iii.	Zwitterion
ii.	Vitamins	iv.	Pathology

b. Give structures of the following:

i.	Lactose	iii.	Ascorbic acid
ii.	Sucrose	iv.	Menadione

c. What is an active site of an enzyme? Explain 'lock and key model' and 'induce fit model'.

d. Explain the role of calcium in our body.

e. Explain the role of following members of cell:

i.	Cell nucleus	iii.	Endoplasmic reticulum
ii.	Cell membrane	iv.	Mitochondria

f. What are fats? Explain rancidity of fats.

g. What are electrolytes? Explain functions of electrolytes in our body.

Q 2. Solve any *three* of the following:

a. Explain ketosis in detail.

b. Explain the terms:

i.	Glycosuria	iii.	Hyperammonaemia
ii.	Glycogenolysis	iv.	Abnormal metabolism

c. Explain 'tricarboxylic acid cycle'.

d. Enlist various functions performed by proteins in our body.

e. Write any *two* identifications test for proteins and denaturation of proteins.

Q 3. Solve any *three* of the following:

a. Write *four* pharmaceutical importance of enzymes.

b. What are polysaccharides? Give their classification with examples and their properties.

   c. Explain the osazone test with reaction.

   d. Differentiate between:

      i. Glucose and fructose

      ii. Peptide linkage and glycosidie linkage

   e. Mention different protein deficiency diseases and explain any *one* of them.

Q 4. Solve any *three* of the following:

   a. What are compound lipids? Classify with examples.

   b. Explain acetyl number and Reichert-Meissel number.

   c. What are phospholipids? Write biological functions of lecithin.

   d. Explain the importance of 'vitamin E'.

   e. What are coenzymes? Name the various vitamins and the coenzymes derived from them.

Q 5. Solve any *three* of the following:

   a. Explain the terms:

      i. Anaemia   ii. Pellagra

   b. Explain the role of 'cyanocobalamin'.

   c. Explain the terms:

      i. Goitre   ii. Polycythemia

   d. Write a note on 'water balance of normal individual'.

   e. Explain the terms:

      i. Purpura   ii. Pyuria

Q 6. Solve any *three* of the following:

   a. What is enzyme inhibition? Explain noncompetitive inhibition.

   b. What is physiological urine and pathological urine?

   c. Explain the role of lymphocytes in health and diseases.

   d. Explain the role of vitamins and minerals in the human body.

   e. Write short note on secondary structure of proteins.

Winter Examination 2008
D Pharm First Year
Biochemistry and Clinical Pathology

Q 1. Solve any *five* of the following.

   a. Define the following terms:

      i. Biochemistry   iii. Anabolism

      ii. Metabolism   iv. Cell

   b. Give structure and biological significance of hyaluronic acid.

   c. Describe the following reactions with their significances:
     i. Molisch's test
     iii. Barfoed's test
     ii. Fehling's test
     iv. Seliwanoff's test
   d. Define proteins. Discuss biological role of proteins.
   e. Explain 'mucosal block theory' of iron absorption.
   f. Give structure and two biological functions of folic acid.
   g. Define physiological urine. Give constituents of physiological urine.

Q 2. Solve any *three* of the following:
   a. Explain the role of blood platelets in coagulation of blood. Give pathology of platelets.
   b. Define the following:
     i. Zymogens
     ii. Cofactors
     iii. Adoptive enzymes
     iv. Constitutive enzymes
   c. Define glycolysis. Give all steps involved in glycolysis, with enzymes and reaction conditions.
   d. Discuss the following reactions of protein catabolism:
     i. Oxidative deamination   ii. Transamination
   e. Explain the structure of starch.

Q 3. Solve any *three* of the following:
   a. Explain the following with example:
     i. Configuration of carbohydrates
     ii. Glycoside linkage
   b. Define amino acids and essential amino acids. Give structure of *two* acidic amino acids.
   c. Discuss biological role of lipids.
   d. What are minerals? Classify them with examples (define each class and subclass).
   e. Define the following:
     i. Anaemia   iii. Haematouria
     ii. Pyuria   iv. Jaundice

Q 4. Solve any *three* of the following:
   a. Explain substrate specificity and reaction specificity of an enzyme.
   b. Define and explain the process of ketogenesis and ketogenolysis.
   c. Discuss the role of lipids in biological membrane with reference to Danielli and Davison model and SJ Singer's model.

    d. Give structures and biological functions of vitamin D.

    e. What is dehydration? Give symptoms and treatment of dehydration.

Q 5. Solve any *three* of the following:

    a. Give *four* points of difference between each of the following:

        i. Competitive inhibition—noncompetitive inhibition.

        ii. Lock and key mechanism—induced fit mechanism.

    b. Explain the following diseases:

        i. Fatty liver   ii. Diabetes mellitus

    c. Give structure and *two* colour reactions of cholesterol.

    d. Describe alpha-helical and beta-pleated structures of proteins.

    e. Explain the factors, affecting absorption of calcium in the body. Give biological functions of calcium.

Q 6. Give steps, in detail, involved in any *three* of the following with enzymes and reaction conditions:

    a. Glycogenesis

    b. Creatine-creatinine pathway

    c. Extramitochondrial fatty acid synthesis

    d. Urea cycle

    e. Krebs cycle

Summer Examination 2009
D Pharm First Year
Biochemistry and Clinical Pathology

Q 1. Solve any *five* of the following.

    a. Name the respective vitamin, nutritional deficiency of which leads to:

        i. Pellagra   iii. Beriberi

        ii. Scurvy   iv. Blood clotting disorder

    b. Define the following:

        i. Sap value   iii. Glycogenesis

        ii. Acid value   iv. Glycogenolysis

    c. Write deficiency diseases of following minerals:

        i. Calcium   iii. Iodine

        ii. Iron   iv. Potassium

    d. Define metabolism, catabolism, anabolism and abnormal metabolism.

    e. Define the following:

        i. Active site of an enzyme   iii. Constitutive enzyme

        ii. Cofactor   iv. Induced enzyme

f. Discuss the different protein deficiency diseases.

g. Define vitamins. Write its classification with examples.

Q 2. Solve any *three* of the following:

a. Define carbohydrate. Write its classification.

b. Define physiological and pathological urine. Write vrious about constituents of urine with their related diseases.

c. Name and write about *two* tests for cholesterol.

d. Define enzyme. Write classification of enzyme.

e. Explain the role of vitamin A in vision.

Q 3. Solve any *three* of the following:

a. Write about osazone test.

b. Write deficiency diseases of lipids.

c. Write classification of protein with example of each.

d.   i. Write various major and trace minerals requried in body.

      ii. Write physiological functions of minerals.

e.   i. Define anaemia. Enumerate different types of anaemia.

      ii. Write about pernicious anaemia.

Q 4. Solve any *three* of following:

a. Define lipids. Write classification of lipids with example.

b. Write the diseases related to carbohydrate metabolism.

c. Enumerate the factors that affect on the rate of catalysed enzyme action. Describe the effect of temperature and pH.

d. Give structure, biological active form, biological function and deficiency disease of vitamin A or thiamine vitamin B_1.

e. Write the therapeutic and pharmaceutical importance of enzyme.

Q 5. Solve any *three* of the following:

a.   i. Define reducing and nonreducing sugars with example.

      ii. Write test and principle of Benedict's test.

b. Write the biological importance of lipids.

c.   i. Define essential and nonessential amino acids with example.

      ii. Enumerate colour tests for proteins.

d. Give structure, biological active form, functions and deficiency disease of niacin.

e. Define enzyme inhibition. Illustrate competitive and noncompetitive inhibition.

Q 6. Solve any *two* of the following:

a. Draw a flow diagram showing the reactions of TCA cycle.

b. Discuss the reactions involved in "urea cycle".

c. Give an account on metabolism of fats with reference to β-oxidation.

Summer Examination 2010
D Pharm First Year
Biochemistry and Clinical Pathology

Q 1. Solve any *five* of the following:

 a. What are biomolecules? Describe the functions of mitochondria.

 b. Give structures of following:

   i. D-Glucose   ii. D-Fructose

   iii. Maltose   iv. Sucrose

 c. Define:

   i. Anabolism   ii. Catabolism

   iii. Metabolism   iv. Gluconeogenesis

 d. What are amino acids? Classify them with suitable examples.

 e. Discuss in short "Denaturation of proteins."

 f. Explain the following:

   i. Anomers   ii. Epimers

 g. Explain the following terms:

   i. Inductive enzyme   ii. Constitutive enzyme

   iii. Zymogens   iv. Isoenzymes

Q 2. Solve any *three*:

 a. Give the classification of carbohydrates with examples.

 b. Discus the diseases related to carbohydrate metabolism.

 c. Give briefly the biological functions of proteins.

 d. What are lymphocytes? Give the different types of lymphocytes.

 e. Discuss in brief the role of lipid.

Q 3. Solve any *three*:

 a. Define lipid. Classify lipids with one example of each class.

 b. Explain the role of phospholipids in biological membrane.

 c. Define and classify vitamins according to thier solubility with examples.

 d. Give the biochemical role of calcium.

 e. Give therapeutic applications of enzymes.

Q 4. Solve any *three*:

 a. Name the factors that affect the velocity of enzymes catalysed reaction. Describe the effect of temperature.

 b. What is E-M pathway? Discuss the various stages of E-M pathway.

 c. Explain the chemical reactions involved in the formation of urea in the body.

 d. Enlist any four abnormal constituents of urine. State their significance.

 e. Explain water balance of normal healthy individual.

Q 5. Solve any *three*:

    a. What are co-enzymes? Name co-enzymes of:

        i. Vitamin B_2 ii. Niacin

    b. Discuss the physiological role and deficiency symptoms of vitamin C.

    c. Discuss in brief the concept of enzyme action.

    d. Describe the primary structure of proteins.

    e. Discuss in brief diabetes mellitus.

Q 6. Solve any *three*:

    a. Explain the following reactions:

        i. Molisch's test   ii. Xanthoprotein test

       iii. Barfoed's test   iv. Biuret test

    b. Define fats and oils. Discuss the physical and chemical properties of fat and oils.

    c. What are minerals? Give in brief their functions.

    d. What is enzyme inhibition? Discuss the different types of enzyme inhibition.

    e. What are abnormalities of red cells? Explain.

Winter Examination 2010
D Pharm First Year
Biochemistry and Clinical Pathology

Q 1. Solve any *eight* of the following:

    a. Define the term "Carbohydrate".

    b. Give the functions of mitochondria.

    c. Give the structure of optically inactive amino acid.

    d. How do fats and oils differ from each other?

    e. Give the symptoms and types of beriberi.

    f. Enlist the B-complex group of vitamins.

    g. Give biological functions of iron.

    h. How water is distributed in the body?

    i. Define the term "Glycosuria" and "Hyperglycemia".

    j. What is meant by "optimum temp" of the enzyme?

    k. What are reducing sugars? Give examples.

    l. Define: Anabolism and catabolism.

Q 2. Solve any *four* of the following:

    a. What are monosaccharides? How they are classified? Give the structure of ketohexose.

    b. What is meant by "Zwitterion"? Explain acid-base behaviour of amino acids.

    c. What are enzymes? How they are classified on the basis of type of reactions catalysed by them.

    d. What is rancidity of fats?

    e. Explain the role of vitamin A in the vision. What are its deficiency syndromes?

    f. Give the diagnostic importance of presence of sugar and ketone bodies in urine.

Q 3. Solve any *four* of the following:

    a. What are homo and hetero-polysaccharides? How do amylose and amylopectin differ from each other?

    b. Explain secondary structures of proteins.

    c. Define lipids. How they are classified? Give examples of each class.

    d. Discuss in brief mechanism of action of enzymes.

    e. Explain the following in brief:

        i. Megaloblastic anemia   ii. Microcytic anemia.

    f. Explain water balance of the body.

Q 4. Solve any *four* of the following:

    a. Give the structures of

        i. Maltose   ii. Lactose

    b. Explain the biological role of calcium in the body.

    c. Explain compective inhibition of enzymes. How it is used to explain mechanism of action of drugs.

    d. What are fatty acids? How they are classified?

    e. Discuss the role of lymphocytes in health and diseases.

    f. Describe animal cell with neat labelled diagram.

Q 5. Solve any *four* of the following:

    a. Explain the following:

        i. Alkaptonuria   ii. Phenylketonuria

    b. Discuss the role of thrombocytes in health diseases.

    c. Explain in brief diagnostic applications of enzymes.

    d. Define the following terms:

        i. Acid value   ii. Saponification value

        iii. Iodine valve

    e. Explain the biochemical role of following co-enzymes.

        i. NAD

        ii. FAD

        iii. TPP

    f. Describe the following in brief:

        i. Pellagra

        ii. Rickets

Q 6. Solve any *four* of the following:
  a. Explain in brief reactions of glycolysis.
  b. What are proteins? How they are classified? What is meant by denaturation of proteins?
  c. Explain transamination and oxidative deamination.
  d. Explain in brief ETC.
  e. Explain in brief reactions of Beta oxidation of fatty acids.
  f. What are phospholipids? Give the structure of lecithin. Explain biological role of phospholipids.

Summer Examination 2011
D Pharm First Year
Biochemistry and Clinical Pathology

Q 1. Solve any *five* of the following:
  a. Explain the terms:
    i. Transamination
    ii. Arteriosclerosis
    iii. Gluconeogenesis
    iv. Metabolism
  b. What is Biochemistry? Mention important organelles of animal cells and their respective functions.
  c. Write the structure for:
    i. D-glucose   ii. D-fructose
    iii. Cholesterol   iv. Nicotinamide
  d. Mention the names of water soluble vitamins and their respective coenzymes.
  e. Define the following:
    i. Compound lipids   ii. Iodine number
    iii. Essential fatty acids   iv. Acid value
  f. What is Pathology? Why are blood and urine sample of a sick person tested? What is the normal composition of blood?
  g. Explain the terms:
    i. Isoenzymes   ii. Marker enzymes
    iii. Egg white injury   iv. Polycythemia

Q 2. Solve any *three* of the following:
  a. Define amino acids and give their classification.
  b. Write short on:
    i. Mutarotation   ii. Starch
  c. What are simple lipids? What is rancidity of fats? Explain the role of antioxidant in preservation of oil.

    d. Explain biochemical functions of vitamin 'A' in detail.

    e. Explain water balance of body.

Q 3. Solve any *three* of the following:

    a. Mention various inborn errors of protein metabolism. Explain 'Alkaptonuria'.

    b. Explain the role of phospholipids in biological membrane with diagram.

    c. Give chemical name of vitamin 'C'. Explain its biochemical role and its deficiency manifestation.

    d. What is enzyme inhibition? Explain competitive inhibition with examples and graph.

    e. What is anemia? Mention different types of anemia. Explain any one of them.

Q 4. Solve any *three* of the following:

    a. Explain the terms:

        i. Peptide bond   ii. Complete proteins

        iii. Protein denaturation   iv. Marasmus

    b. Explain the identification test for each

        i. Carbohydrates   ii. Proteins

    c. What are enzymes? Give their classification.

    d. What is meant by Physiological Urine and Pathological Urine? Mention abnormal constituents of urine and their significance.

    e. What are Minerals? Give their functions in biological system.

Q 5. Solve any *three* of the following:

    a. State and explain qualitative tests for proteins.

    b. Define vitamins and explain the terms

        i. Rickets   ii. Beriberi

    c. What are carbohydrates? Give their biological importance. Mention names of commonly consumed carbohydrates.

    d. What is an active site of an enzyme? Explain 'Lock and key model' and 'Induce fit model' with diagram.

    e. Explain the terms:

        i. Goitre

        ii. Hyponatremia

        iii. Osteoporosis

        iv. Electrolytes

Q 6. Solve any *two* of the following:

    a. Explain biosynthesis of urea.

    b. Explain glycolysis

    c. Explain β-oxidation of fatty acids.

Winter Examination 2011
D Pharm First Year
Biochemistry and Clinical Pathology

Q 1. Solve any *five* of the following:

   a. Define the term 'Biochemistry' with scope.

   b. Give structures of the following:

i. D-glucose	ii. Niacin
iii. Pyridoxin	iv. D-Mannose

   c. Explain the primary structure of protein.

   d. Explain the role of Phospholipids in biological membrane.

   e. Give the importance of minerals in biological system.

   f. Define the following terms:

i. Co-enzyme	ii. Co-factor

   g. What do you mean by:

i. Metabolism	ii. Anabolism
iii. Catabolism	iv. Gluconeogenesis

Q 2. Solve any three of the following:

   a. Give the principle involved in:

i. Molish's test	ii. Millon's test

   b. Give the classification of carbohydrates with examples.

   c. Define the following terms:

i. Saponification value	ii. Acetyl valve
iii. Iodine value	iv. Acid valve

   d. Classify vitamins according to their solubility with examples.

   e. What is Kerbs cycle? State briefly the steps of Kerbs cycle.

Q 3. Solve any *three* of the following:

   a. Give therapeutic importance of enzyme.

   b. What are abnormalities of red cells? Explain.

   c. What is phenylketonuria? Discuss the pathway of phenylketonuria.

   d. Give the classification of lipids with example.

   e. What are the diseases occurred due to disorders of lipid metabolism?

Q 4. Solve any *three* of the following:

   a. Give absorption, excretion and functions of vitamin D.

   b. Mention different factors affecting enzyme catalysed reaction. What is the effect of temperature on it?

   c. What is biochemical role of calcium?

   d. Explain the chemical reactions involved in the formation of urea in the body.

  e. What are the normal organic and inorganic constituents of urine? Describe.

Q 5. Solve any *three* of the following:

  a. What are Proteins? Give their biological function.
  b. Discuss in brief the concept of enzyme action.
  c. Explain the following reactions:
    i. Ninhydrine test
    ii. Fehling test
    iii. Benedict's test
    iv. Emulsification test
  d. Discuss in short the distribution of water in body and its functions.
  e. Name the respective vitamin, nutritional deficiency of which leads to:
    i. Xerophthalmia
    ii. Pellagra
    iii. Hemorrhage
    iv. Beriberi
    v. Pernicious anemis
    vi. Scurvy

Q 6. Solve any *two* of the following:

  a. Discuss the reactions involved in β-oxidation.
  b. What is E-M pathway? Discuss the various stages of E-M pathway.
  c. i. Define Proteinuria and Glycosuria
     ii. What is Transamination? Discuss.

Summer Examination 2012
D Pharm First Year
Biochemistry and Clinical Pathology

Q 1. Solve any *five* of the following:

  a. Give structure and two important functions of:
    i. Mitochondria
    ii. Endoplasmic reticulum
  b. Explain classification of carbohydrates giving examples and defining each term.
  c. Give Osazone formation test and its significance.
  d. Discuss acid-base nature of amino acids and explain isoelectric point of amino acid.
  e. Define the following in relation of lipids:
    i. Acid value
    ii. Saponification value
    iii. Iodine value
    iv. Reichert Meissel value
  f. Give structure and two colour reactions of cholesterol.
  g. Give biological role of iron in human body (explain any *four* detail).

Q 2. Solve any *three* of the following:

    a. Give name of co-enzyme and its one biological functions of the following vitamins:

        i. Thiamine hydrochloride   ii. Pyridoxin

       iii. Riboflavin   iv. Nicotinamide

    b. Explain causes, symptoms and treatment for dehydration.

    c. Explain secondary structure of proteins.

    d. Define anemia. Explain megaloblastic and sickle cell anemia.

    e. Explain the following terms:

        i. Adoptive enzymes

       ii. Constitutive enzymes

      iii. Isoenzymes

      iv. Allosteric enzymes

Q 3. Solve any *three* of the following:

    a. Explain four pharmaceutical and therapeutic uses of enzymes.

    b. Explain the following:

        i. Coris cycle

       ii. Mucosal block theory of iron absorption.

    c. Define the following:

        i. Enzymes

       ii. One unit of enzyme activity

      iii. Turnover number of enzymes

      iv. Specific activity of enzymes

    d. Define Glycolysis. Explain all steps involved in glycolysis.

    e. Define pathological urine. Give significance of any three abnormal constituents of urine.

Q 4. Solve any *three* of the following:

    a. What is enzyme inhibition? Give six points of difference between competitive inhibition of non-competitive inhibition.

    b. Explain the structure of starch.

    c. Give and explain two protein deficiency diseases.

    d. What are glycolipids? Give its structure.

    e. Explain in detail any four factors affecting absorption of calcium.

Q 5. Solve any *three* of the following:

    a. Give structure and biological role of vitamin 'A' in relation to vision (eye).

    b. Explain water balance in human body (give definition, outgoing and incoming sources and account of water).

    c. Discuss role of lipids in biological membrane with the help of models.

   d. Enlist factors affecting rate of enzyme catalysed reaction. Explain in detail effect of substrate concentration with the help and curves and equations.

   e. Give the following reaction:
      i. Seliwanoff's reaction
      ii. Biuret reaction
      iii. Ninhydrin reaction
      iv. Saponification reaction.

Q 6. Solve any *three* of the following:

(Give only steps with reaction conditions)
   a. β-oxidation of fatty acids
   b. Krebs cycle
   c. Urea cycle
   d. Creatine-Creatinine pathway
   e. Glycogenesis.

Winter Examination 2012
D Pharm First Year
Biochemistry and Clinical Pathology

Q 1. Solve any *five* of the following:
   a. What are carbohydrates? Give its classification.
   b. Give pharmaceutical and therapeutic significance of enzymes.
   c. Explain the role of vitamin 'A' in vision.
   d. What are proteins? Give biological importance of proteins.
   e. Explain the role of lipids in biological membrane
   f. Explain mutarotation with example.
   g. Explain the role of platelets in health and disease.

Q 2. Solve any *three* of the following:
   a. Explain the following:
      i. Rickets
      ii. Beriberi
   b. Define the following:
      i. Co-factor
      ii. Constitutive enzymes
      iii. Co-enzymes
      iv. Marker enzymes
   c. Give the structures of:
      i. Sucrose   ii. Lactose

d. Define the following terms:
    i. Saponification value
    ii. Reichert-Meissel number
e. Define biochemistry. Give its importance.

Q 3. Solve any *three* of the following:

a. Define the following terms:
    i. Metabolism   ii. Anabolism
    iii. Prokaryotic cell   iv. Eukaryotic cell
b. Explain water balance in human body.
c. What are lipids? Give functions of lipids.
d. Explain the formation of Osazone of maltose and lactose.
e. What are triglycerides? Give its functions.

Q 4. Solve any *three* of the following:

a. Give the structure of:
    i. Cholesterol   ii. Isoprenoid unit
    iii. Progesterone   iv. Androsterone
b. Give functions of vitamin 'C'.
c. Give name of co-enzymes of the following vitamins:
    i. Riboflavin   ii. Pentothenic acid
    iii. Cynocobalamine   iv. Folic acid
d. Explain the following:
    i. Megaloblastic anaemia
    ii. Sickle cell anemia
e. Explain acid-base behaviour of amino acid.

Q 5. Solve any *three* of the following:

a. What happen when amino acid react with
    i. 1 Fluoro-2, 4, dinitro benzene (FDNB)
    ii. Formaldehyde
b. Explain complete and incomplete proteins with examples.
c. Explain the following in brief:
    i. Kwashiorkar   ii. Marasmus
d. What are peptides and polypeptides?
e. Explain biochemical role and deficiency symptoms of:
    i. Iron
    ii. Zinc

Q 6. Solve any *two* of the following:

a. Explain in brief reactions involved in Glycolysis.
b. Give the steps of Kerbs cycle and its energetics.
c. Explain 'β' oxidation of fatty acid.

Summer Examination 2013
D Pharm First Year
Biochemistry and Clinical Pathology

Q 1. Solve any *five* of the following:

    a. Define following terms:

        i. Saponification value   ii. Acetyl value

        iii. Iodine value   iv. Acid value

    b. Give structure of the following:

        i. Niacin   ii. Sucrose

        iii. D-glucose   iv. Ascorbic acid

    c. Explain the following terms:

        i. Co-enzymes   ii. Co-factor

        iii. Zymogens   iv. Inductive enzymes

    d. Explain any four roles of iron in human body.

    e. What are amino acids? Classify them with suitable examples.

    f. Explain following reactions:

        i. Barfoed's test   ii. Biuret test

        iii. Fehlings test   iv. Emulsification test

    g. Give osazone formation test and its significance.

Q 2. Solve any *three* of the following:

    a. Explain the secondary structure of protein.

    b. Define carbohydrates and classify them with examples.

    c. Discuss in short distribution of water in body and its functions.

    d. Explain various functions performed by protein in our body.

    e. Explain the terms:

        i. Haematuria   ii. Ketoacidosis

        iii. Gluconeogenesis   iv. Anabolism

Q 3. Solve any *three* of the following:

    a. Name the factors that affect velocity of the enzyme catalysed reaction. Describe effect of temperature.

    b. Name the respective vitamin, nutritional deficiency of which leads to:

        i. Blood clotting disorders   ii. Beriberi

        iii. Night blindness   iv. Pellagra

    c. Define anemia. Enumerate different types of anemia. Explain pernicious anemia.

    d. Discuss different protein deficiency diseases.

    e. What are the lymphocytes? Classify them. Give two important functions of lymphocytes.

Q 4. Solve any *three* of the following:

a. Define fats and oils. Discuss physical and chemical properties of fats and oils.

b. Give structure; biological active form, biological functions and deficiency diseases of vitamin D.

c. Discuss in brief role of lipids.

d. Explain causes, symptoms and treatment for dehydration.

e. Name and explain two test for cholesterol.

Q 5. Solve any *three* of the following:

a. Discuss in brief "Glycolysis".

b. Describe typical cell with neat labelled diagram.

c. Explain applications of enzyme.

d. Write various major and trance minerals required in body. Write physiological functions of minerals.

e. Define enzyme inhibition. Explain competitive and non-competitive inhibition.

Q 6. Solve any *two* of the following:

a. Draw a flow diagram showing the reaction of Kerbs cycle. Give energetics.

b. Explain β-oxidation of fats in details.

c. Explain in brief "Urea Cycle".

d. Explain electron transport and respiratory chain.

Winter Examination 2013
D Pharm First Year
Biochemistry and Clinical Pathology

Q 1. Solve any *five* of the following:

a. Draw a neat labelled diagram of typical cell and describe functions of nucleus.

b. Give the structure of following:
   i. D-Galactose
   ii. D-Fructose
   iii. Lactose
   iv. Sucrose

c. Explain the following terms.
   i. Zymogen
   ii. Isoenzyme
   iii. Metalloenzyme
   iv. Allosteric enzyme

    d. What do you mean by "zwitter ion"? Explain acid-base behaviour of amino acid.

    e. Define following:
       i. Sap value   ii. Acid value
      iii. Glycogenesis   iv. Gluconeogenesis

    f. Explain 'Lock and Key Model' and 'Induced Fit Model' of enzyme action.

    g. Explain deficiency disorders of protein.

Q 2. Solve any *three* of the following:

    a. Explain osazone formation of carbohydrate. Give its significance.

    b. Give diagnostic and therapeutic applications of enzyme.

    c. Give physiological role of iodine.

    d. Explain the following:
       i. Essential fatty acids with example
      ii. Rancidification of fats and oils.

    e. Name the vitamins of which deficiency leads to:
       i. Pellagra   ii. Scurvy
      iii. Beriberi   iv. Blood clotting disorder
       v. Rickets   vi. Night blindness
     vii. Pernicious anemia   viii. Egg white injury

Q 3. Solve any *three* of the following:

    a. Define carbohydrates and classify them with examples.

    b. What are co-enzymes? Name the co-enzymes of vitamins B_2 and B_3.

    c. Explain water balance of normal individual.

    d. What are lymphocytes? Give their role in health and diseases.

    e. Give the structure and colour reactions of cholesterol.

Q 4. Solve any *three* of the following:

    a. Explain role of vitamin A in vision cycle.

    b. Mention the factors affecting rate of enzyme catalysed reactions. Explain effect of temperature and pH on enzyme catalysed reaction.

    c. i. Differentiate between reducing and non-reducing sugars.
      ii. Write the test and principle of Molisch's test.

    d. Give the biological importance of lipids.

    e. Write physiological functions of minerals.

Q 5. Solve any *three* of the following:

    a. Define enzyme and classify them with example.

    b. What is pathological urine? Name abnormal constituents of urine with the ailment associated with them.

    c. Give the following reactions of amino acids with their significance:
       i. Ninhydrin reaction   ii. FDNB reaction

d. Give the structure and functions of vitamins B_1 or B_6.

e. How will you detect the following from the given sample of urine:

    i. Sugar   ii. Blood

Q 6. Solve any *two* of the following:

a. Draw a flow diagram showing the reactions of TCA cycle.

b. Explain 'Urea Cycle'.

c. Give an account of metabolism of fats with reference to β-oxidation.

Winter Examination 2014
D Pharm First Year
Biochemistry and Clinical Pathology

Q 1. Attempt any *five* of the following:

a. Define the following:

    i. Ketosis   ii. Glycosuria

    iii. Polyuria   iv. Purpura.

b. Explain the role of following members of cell:

    i. Cell nucleus   ii. Cell membrane

    iii. Mitochondria   iv. Endoplasmic reticulum.

c. Explain the rancidification of fats:

d. Give the structures of followings:

    i. D-Glucose   ii. D-Frutose

    iii. Menadione   iv. Ascorbic acid.

e. What are the reducing and non reducing sugars? Give examples.

f. Define co-enzymes:

    i. Folic acid   ii. Pyridoxine

    iii. Cyanocobalamin

g. Explain the structure of starch.

Q 2. Attempt any *three* of the following:

a. Define lipids give the classification with example

b. Explain denaturation of proteins

c. Give the following reactions of amino acids with their significance:

    i. Ninhydrin reaction

    ii. Reaction with dansyl chloride

d. Explain epimer and anomer with suitable example

e. Give the structure and two color reaction of cholesterol

Q 3. Attempt any *three* of the following:

a. Explain secondary structure of proteins.

b. What is an active site of enzyme? Explain lock model and key model and induced fit model.

    c. Explain biological importance and absorption iron

    d. Explain the following reaction:
       i. Biuret test
      ii. Xanthoprotic test
     iii. Seliwanoff's test
     iv. Molisch's test

    e. Enumerate the factor that affects the rate of enzyme catalyzed reaction. Describe the effect of temperature and PH.

Q 4. Attempt any *three* of the following:

    a. Discuss the following reactions of protein catabolism:
       i. Oxidative deamination
      ii. Transamination

    b. Define and classify minerals give the functions of minerals.

    c. Define physiological and pathological urine write various abnormal constituents of urine with their related disease.

    d. Explain:
       i. Microcytic anemia
      ii. Diabetes mellitus

    e. Discuss the different protein deficiency disease.

Q 5. Attempt any *three* of the following:

    a. Define the following:
       i. Anabolism   ii. Acetyl number
     iii. Isoenzymes   iv. Anuria

    b. Define enzyme and classification of enzyme.

    c. Explain the biochemical role of calcium and factors affecting rate of absorption of calcium in body

    d. What the phospholipids? Give the biological importance and structure of any one phospholipid.

    e. Discuss in brief any two of following:
       i. Egg white injury
      ii. Scurvy
     iii. Pellagra

Q 6. Attempt any *three* of the following:

    a. Discuss the reaction involved in urea cycle.

    b. Explain all steps involved in glycolysis.

    c. Give the reaction involved in Krebs cycle.

    d. Define and classify amino acids with examples write structure of any one sulphur containing amino acids.

    e. Explain β-oxidation of fatty acids.

Summer Examination 2015
D Pharm First Year
Biochemistry and Clinical Pathology

Q 1. Solve any *five* of the following:

  a. Define the following:
     i. Metabolism
     ii. Abnormal metabolism
     iii. Catabolism
     iv. Anabolism
  b. What is an active site of an enzyme and explain 'Lock & Key Model' and 'Induced fit Model'?
  c. Explain acid-base behaviour of amino acids.
  d. Define and classify carbohydrates with examples.
  e. Explain the role of vitamin A in vision.
  f. Discuss biochemical role of calcium and diseases caused by calcium deficiency.
  g. Define following terms with examples:
     i. Epimers
     ii. Anomers

Q 2. Solve any *three* of the following:

  a. Define and classify vitamins with examples. Name the vitamins belongs to B-complex group.
  b. Explain water balance of normal individual.
  c. Enlist and explain different protein deficiency diseases.
  d. Discuss following reactions of monosaccharides:
     i. Osazone formation
     ii. Oxidation
  e. Enumerate the factors affecting rate of enzyme catalysed reaction.
  f. Discuss in detail effect of enzyme concentration and effect of temperature.

Q 3. Solve any *three* of the following:

  a. Give physiological functions, deficiency symptoms and structure of niacin.
  b. Define:
     i. Acid value
     ii. Saponification value
     iii. Iodine number
     iv. Reichert-Meissl number

   c. What are electrolytes? Give functions of electrolytes in our body.

   d. Name the respective vitamin responsible for nutritional deficiency cause:
    i. Osteoporosis
    ii. Blood clotting disorder
    iii. Beriberi
    iv. Night blindness
    v. Pernicious anaemia
    vi. Scurvy
    vii. Rickets
    viii. Egg white injury

   e. Draw a neat labelled diagram of typical animal cell. Give functions of mitochondria and nucleus.

Q 4. Solve any *three* of the following:

   a. What are abnormal constituents of urine ? Give their significance in diseases.

   b. Define and classify ammo acids by giving suitable examples.

   c. Give the structures of following:
    i. D-Glucose
    ii. Fructose
    iii. Galactose
    iv. Mannose

   d. Give structure and colour reactions of cholesterol.

   e. Differentiate between competitive and non-competitive enzyme inhibition.

Q 5. Solve any *three* of the following:

   a. Define:
    i. Endoenzyme
    ii. Exoenzyme
    iii. Induced enzyme
    iv. Isoenzymes

   b. Explain biological functions of proteins.

   c. Define anaemia. Enlist different types of anaemia. Explain aplastic anaemia and megaloblastic anaemia.

   d. Explain the following:
    i. Essential fatty acids
    ii. Non-essential fatty acids

   e. How acetone and sugar are detected in urine?

Q 6. Solve any *three* of the following:

   a. Explain in brief reactions involved in TC A cycle.

   b. Give an account of metabolism of fats with reference to β-oxidation.

   c. Explain formation of urea in body.

   d. Explain reactions involved in glycolysis.

   e. Describe the following :
      i. Benedict's test
      ii. Barfoed's test
      iii. Fehlings test
      iv. Saliwanoff's test

Winter Examination 2015
D Pharm First Year
Biochemistry and Clinical Pathology

Q 1. Attempt any *eight* of the following:

   a. Define 'Bio-chemistry' and state its significance in pharmacy.

   b. Draw a neat labelled diagram of mitochondria and describe its functions.

   c. Give structures of:
      i. D-Glucose
      ii. Sucrose

   d. What are essential amino acids? Enlist any four of them.

   e. Explain the following terms:
      i. Glycogenesis
      ii. Gluconeogenesis

   f. Write following tests of carbohydrates:
      i. Benedict's test
      ii. Molisch's test

   g. What is 'anaemia'? Describe 'sickle-cell' anaemia.

   h. Explain the following:
      i. Metabolism
      ii. Pathological urine

   i. Enlist fat soluble vitamins.

   j. Distinguish between fats and oils.

   k. What are minerals? Give their biochemical functions (any **four**).

   l. What is meant by 'marker enzymes'?

Q 2. Attempt any *four* of the following:

   a. Define and classify 'carbohydrates'.

   b. Write biological functions of proteins.

   c. What are compound lipids? Give their classification with suitable examples.

    d. Explain the following terms:
       i. Lecithines
      ii. Rancidity
    e. Mention the names of water soluble vitamins and their respective co-enzymes.
    f. How will you identify following constituents in the given sample of urine:
       i. Ketone bodies
      ii. Proteins
     iii. Blood

Q 3. Attempt any *four* of the following:

    a. Explain the following:
       i. Alkaptonuria
      ii. Phenylketonuria
    b. What are enzymes? Give their classifications.
    c. Explain water balance of body.
    d. What is enzyme inhibition? Explain competitive inhibition with example.
    e. Write structure and give two biochemical functions of Vit. B_1.
    f. Describe alpha-helical and beta-pleated structures of proteins.

Q 4. Attempt any *four* of the following:

    a. Enlist factors affecting rate of enzyme catalysed reaction. Explain effect of temperature.
    b. Define the following:
       i. Jaundice
      ii. Pyaria
     iii. Haematouria
    c. Give structure and two colour reactions of cholesterol.
    d. Draw structure and give biological functions of vit. D.
    e. What is dehydration? Write symptoms and treatment of dehydration.
    f. Explain factors affecting absorption of calcium in the body. Give biochemical functions of calcium.

Q 5. Attempt any *four* of the following:

    a. Explain the following terms:
       i. Allosteric enzyme
      ii. Purpura
    b. Explain role of vit. A in vision.
    c. Define the following terms and give their significance:
       i. Acid value
      ii. Iodine value
     iii. Saponification value

d. Describe the following in brief:
   i. Pellagra
   ii. Rickets
e. What are 'Lymphocytes'? Discuss their role in health and disease.
f. What is ketosis? Enlist ketone bodies.

Q 6. Attempt any *four* of the following:
a. Explain in brief reactions of Glycolysis.
b. Define the following:
   i. Induced enzymes
   ii. Isoenzymes
   iii. Zymogens
c. Explain the following:
   i. Metarotation
   ii. Epigerism
d. Discuss in brief 'Denaturation' of proteins.
e. Explain in brief reactions of urea cycle.
f. Explain in brief reactions of beta-oxidation of fatty acids.

Summer Examination 2016
D Pharm First Year
Biochemistry and Clinical Pathology

Q 1. Solve any *eight* of the following :
a. Define the following terms:
   i. Iodine value
   ii. Saponification value
b. Explain the following terms:
   i. Glycogenesis
   ii. Gluconeogenesis
c. Define and classify 'Vitamins'.
d. Give biochemical functions and deficiency manifestations of Iodine.
e. What are co-enzymes ? Name co-enzymes derived from:
   i. Vitamin Bp
   ii. Vitamin B_3
f. Distinguish between Fats and Oils.
g. What are reducing sugars? Give suitable examples.
h. Enlist any four essential amino acids.
i. Define the term 'Biochemistry'. State its importance in pharmacy.
j. What happens when glucose is oxidised and reduced?

    k. Define:
        i. Anabolism
        ii. Catabolism
    l. Give functions of
        i. Mitochondria
        ii Endoplasmic reticulum

Q 2. Solve any *four* of the following:

    a. Define and classify carbohydrates.
    b. Write structures of:
        i. Glucose
        ii. Fructose
        iii. Lactose
        iv. Sucrose
    c. Explain the following terms:
        i. Mutarotation
        ii. Epimerism
    d. Explain role of lipids in biological membrane.
    e. What are proteins? Classify them with suitable examples.
    f. Write any four biochemical functions of proteins.

Q 3. Solve any *four* of the following:

    a. What is meant by:
        i. Thermal denaturation
        ii. Rancidity
    b. Explain the following terms:
        i. Egg white injury
        ii. Hypervitaminosis
    c. Describe in brief role of Vit. A in vision.
    d. Define and classify lipids.
    e. Write in brief about
        i. Transamination
        ii. Oxidative deamination
    f. Give pharmaceutical and therapeutic significance of enzymes.

Q 4. Solve any *four* of the following:

    a. Explain enzyme binding of a substrate with the help of suitable models.
    b. What are lymphocytes? Explain their role in health and disease.
    c. Explain water balance of the adult healthy individual.
    d. Write biochemical role and deficiency symptoms of:
        i. Calcium
        ii. Zinc

  e. Explain in brief the following terms:
    i. Kwashiorkor
    ii. Marasmus
  f. Give functions of Vit. C.

Q 5. Solve any *four* of the following:

  a. What is anaemia? Write in brief about sickle cell anaemia.
  b. Draw a neat and well labelled diagram of typical animal cell.
  c. What are electrolytes? Write functions of electrolytes.
  d. Enlist various factors affecting rate of enzyme catalysed reaction. Explain in detail role of temperature.
  e. Define the following terms:
    i. Exoenzymes
    ii. Endoenzymes
    iii. Induced enzymes
    iv. Zymogens
  f. Give functions of folic acid.

Q 6. Solve any *four* of the following:

  a. What is ATP? What is its role in biological system?
  b. Explain the following terms:
    i. Ketosis
    ii. Pellagra
  c. Explain in brief reactions of glycolysis.
  d. What is dehydration? Give its symptoms and treatment. Write role of ORS.
  e. Explain in brief reactions of urea cycle.
  f. What are enzyme? How are they classified on the basis of types of reaction catalysed by them?

Winter Examination 2016
D Pharm First Year
Biochemistry and Clinical Pathology

Q 1. Solve any *eight* of the following:

  a. What is biochemistry?
  b. Define cell and give functions of cell membrane.
  c. Distinguish between reducing and non-reducing sugars.
  d. Give the structure of glycine.
  e. Define anabolism and catabolism.
  f. What are co-enzymes?
  g. Give symptoms due to deficiency of Vit. C.

    h. What is osteoporosis?

    i. Differentiate between fats and oils.

    j. Define the term—Holoenzyme and apoenzyme.

    k. How sugar and blood is detected in urine sample?

    1. Define—Pyuria and Haematuria.

Q 2. Solve any *four* of the following:

    a. Define following: (any **three**)

        i. Sap value

        ii. Acid value

        iii. Polensky number

        iv. Iodine number

    b. Define carbohydrate and classify them with examples.

    c. What do you mean by "Zwitterion". Explain acid-base behaviour of amino acid.

    d. Explain 'Lock and Key Model' of enzyme action.

    e. Explain water balance of normal individual.

    f. What is pathological urine? Name four abnormal constituents with their significance.

Q 3. Solve any *four* of the following:

    a. Explain role of Vit. A in vision cycle.

    b. Define enzymes; classify them with examples.

    c. Explain primary structure of protein.

    d. Give reaction of following reagents with amino acids—

        i. FDNB

        ii. Ninhydrin

    e. Write short account of:

        i. Beriberi

        ii. Pellagra

    f. What are lymphocytes? Give their role in health and disease.

Q 4. Solve any *four* of the following:

    a. Explain 'Mutarotation' of D-glucose.

    b. Give structure and colour reactions of cholesterol

    c. Explain following:

        i. Essential fatty acids with examples.

        ii. Rancidification of fats and oils.

    d. Name the vitamins, deficiency of which leads to:

        i. Egg white injury

        ii. Pernicious anaemia

        iii. Scurvy

        iv. Night blindness

     v. Rickets

    vi. Blood clotting disorder

  e. What is dehydration? Give symptoms and treatment of dehydration.

  f. Explain the term phenylketoneuria and Maple syrup urine disease.

Q 5. Solve any *four* of the following:

  a. Mention factors affecting rate of enzyme catalysed reaction. Discuss effect of temperature and pH on enzyme catalysed reaction.

  b. Write physiological functions of minerals.

  c. Give the structure of D-glucose; D-fructose and D-galactose.

  d. Define (any **three**):

    i. Isoenzyme

    ii. Multienzyme

    iii. Constitutive enzyme

    iv. Zymogen

  e. Explain the biochemical role of followihg co-enzyme:

    i. NAD

    ii. FAD

    iii. TPP

  f. What are vitamins? Classify with examples.

Q 6. Solve any *four* of the following:

  a. Give steps involved in glycolysis with enzymes.

  b. Discuss following reactions with importance

    i. Transamination and

    ii. Oxidative deamination

  c. Discuss in brief the reactions involved in β-oxidation of fatty acids.

  d. Discuss energetics of TCA cycle.

  e. Explain the structure of starch.

  f. Give biological functions of phospholipids and write structure of any phospholipid.

Summer Examination 2017
D Pharm First Year
Biochemistry and Clinical Pathology

Q 1. Solve any *eight* of the following:

  a. Define Biochemistry. State the importance in pharmacy.

  b. Give functions of mitochondria and endoplasmic reticulum.

  c. Give the structure of optically inactive amino acid and any one aromatic amino acid.

    d. What is non-reducing sugar? Give suitable examples.
    e. Give the structure of D-fructose and D-mannose.
    f. Differentiate between peptide linkage and glycosidic linkage.
    g. Define essential and non-essential fatty acid with example.
    h. Give symptoms due to deficiency of ascorbic acid
    i. What are co-enzymes and name coenzymes derived from (i) Vitamin B_1 and (b) Vitamin B_3?
    j. Define and classify vitamin.
    k. Give biological functions of calcium.
    l. Write deficiency disease of iron and potassium.

Q 2. Solve any *four* of the following:
    a. Define and classify ainino acid with examples.
    b. Define protein. Mention biological functions of proteins.
    c. Define and classify carbohydrates with examples.
    d. Explain rhodopsin cycle for vision.
    e. Explain water balance of normal individual.
    f. Discuss diagnostic and therapeutic applications of enzymes.

Q 3. Solve any *four* of the following:
    a. Explain α-helix structure of protein.
    b. Explain acid-base behaviour of amino acids.
    c. Explain mutarotation with example.
    d. Give the structure, biochemical role and deficiency disease of nicotinic acid.
    e. Explain the mucosal block theory of iron absorption.
    f. What is physiological and pathological urine? Mention abnormal constituents of urine and their significance in disease.

Q 4. Solve any *four* of the following:
    a. Explain following reactions:
        i. Biuret test
        ii. Ninhydrine test
        iii. Xanthoproteic test
    b. Explain the osazone reaction of carbohydrate with its significance.
    c. Explain the following term with their significance.
        i. Acid value
        ii. Iodine value
    d. Name the vitamin deficiency of which leads to:
        i. Beriberi
        ii. Egg white injury
        iii. Rickets

    iv. Pernicious anaemia

    v. Scurvy

    vi. Blood clotting disorder

  e. Define enzyme and classify enzymes with examples.

  f. What are abnormalities of red cells? Explain.

Q 5. Solve any *four* of the following:

  a. Explain the diseases caused by dietary deficiency of proteins.

  b. Describe glycogen storage disease and diabetes mellitus.

  c. Explain the role of lipids in biological membrane.

  d. What are electrolytes? Explain functions of electrolytes in our body.

  e. What is enzyme inhibition? Explain competitive and non competitive inhibition with examples.

  f. What are lymphocytes? Explain role of lymphocytes in health and diseases.

Q 6. Solve any *four* of the following:

  a. What is E-M pathway? Give steps involved in E-M pathway.

  b. Discuss TCA cycle along with its energetics.

  c. Explain the urea cycle.

  d. Discuss Beta-oxidation by taking example of palmitic acid.

  e. Define:

    i. Iso-enzyme

    ii. Multienzyme

    iii. Allosteric enzymes

    iv. Metallo enzymes

  f. What are lipids? Classify lipids with examples. Give one structure of unsaturated fatty acid.